LIVING proof

LIVING
proof
Is there a cure for cancer?

John Cirocco

mg

Published by
Margaret Gee
PO Box 221, Double Bay NSW 1360, Australia
Tel: (02) 9365 3266   Fax: (02) 9365 3168

With sincere thanks to Brian Ansell
who introduced the Publisher to this book

First published 1997
Second edition 2000

National Library of Australia Cataloguing-in-Publication entry
Cirocco, John, 1963-
Living proof: is there a cure for cancer?

ISBN 1 875574 36 0

Design and print management
Reno Design Group, Sydney   R19145
Designer
Graham Rendoth
Photography
Courtesy of John Cirocco
Printing
McPherson's Printing Group
Distribution
Gary Allen Pty Ltd
Typesetting
Berkeley, Frutiger Condensed

5 4 3 2 1

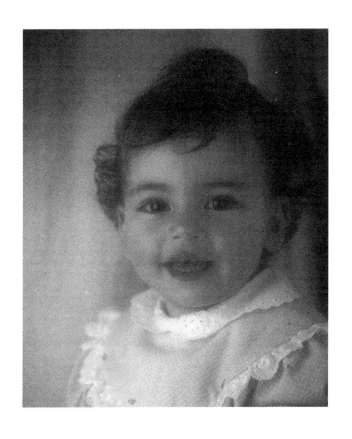

IN MEMORY OF *LAURA*
YOU TAUGHT ME TO FEAR NOT

DISCLAIMER

The information, procedure and suggestions contained in this book are based on the research and the personal experiences of the author.

They are not intended to replace the services of a licensed medical doctor. The author himself is not a medical doctor and does not purport to offer medical advice, make diagnoses, prescribe remedies for specific medical conditions or substitute for medical consultation.

The publisher and author are not responsible for any adverse effects or consequences resulting from the use of any of the suggestions, preparations or procedures discussed in this book.

Consultation with your doctor is recommended prior to adopting any of the treatments set forth in this book.

DEDICATION

I would like to dedicate this book to my wife Anna. Without her I would never have come this far. To my children who are our future and fill every day of our life with love and laughter. To all our dear and special friends we met in Mexico who inspired me to write this book.

May this book give hope and inspiration to all who seek it. May it be a guide to help find the answer you are looking for.

I would strongly urge anyone about to undergo surgery, radiation or chemotherapy to read this book.

"But nobody can say that one does not know what cancer and its prime cause can be. On the contrary, there is no disease whose prime cause is better known, so that today ignorance is no excuse that one cannot do more about prevention. That prevention of cancer will come there is no doubt, for man wishes to survive. But how long prevention will be avoided depends on how long the prophets of agnosticism will succeed in inhibiting the application of scientific knowledge in the cancer field. In the meantime, millions of people must die of cancer unnecessarily."

OTTO WARBURG, dual Nobel Prize Laureate, 1966

ACKNOWLEDGMENTS

From conception to completion, this book has taken over two years of research and discussion with hundreds of cancer patients. I especially wish to acknowledge the following:

- *Charlotte Gerson*, who inspired me to not only believe in myself but to also share my victory with others. Your father's spirit lives within me! Thank you Charlotte.

- Our dear *friends in Mexico* who encouraged us to tell our story to the world.

- *Anna*, my dedicated wife. Without her untiring positive input, I could not have regained my health or completed this book. Thank you sweetheart!

- To our wonderful, supportive parents. *Frank & Litz*, and *Pat & Lisa*.

- A very special thanks to *Rick Sobaszek, David Baldichinno, Jeff & Barbara Blanco* for their wonderful support when I most needed it.

- *Robert Roddy*, who translated my innermost thoughts into words. Along with his emotion and intellect, he brilliantly captured the essence of our story.

- *Kathryn Alexander*, who helped us in the final stages of this book. Thank you Kathryn, you are a true inspiration!

- All our dear *friends* and *family* who have supported us unconditionally.

- Our children, who motivated me to write this book. Thank you *Olivia*, *Christian* and *Lawrence*, I love you.

I wish to sincerely thank the following people for their generous support. Without their assistance, the original edition of this book could not have been published. Thank you.

Neil & Annette Anderson
David Baldichinno
Frank & Italia Barilla
Jeff & Barbara Blanco
Peter & Ada Blanco
Angelo & Mario Boffa
Michael & Susan Bowman
Samuel & Victoria Bowman
Tony Cabarrus
Steven & Diana Capaldo
Stephen & Jo Chambers
Rocco & Antonia Cirocco
Tony & Rosie Cirocco
Tony & Geraldine De Conno
Michael De Ieso
Ralph & Livvy
  Di Benedetto
Stephen & Rosie Edwards
Mario & Gina Emanuele
Robert & Yolanda Fragomeni
Ennio & Joanne Frocione
Marco & Koula Giannini

Matt Goodlet
Peter & Kay Greig
Martin Haese
John Henderson
Charlie & Adele Ielasi
Sean Kay
(In memory of Jim Kay)
George & Joanna Kavaleros
Roger Kozuch
George Mallios
Stuart & Julie Marshall
David & Diedre McLaren
Doug & Betty Mackenzie
Greg & Sonya Perks
Harry & Carol Perks
Rocky Perre
Ross Perre
Mark & Patricia Perre
Gordon Pickard
Bruno & Rita Piteo
Max & Lyn Prince
Sam & Tass Raptopoulos
Ellen Roddy
Mark & Kirsty Roderick

Dean Santin
Gilbert Saupin
Mando & Julianne Scarsella
John & Robert Silvestri
Rick Sobaszek
John Smania
Andrew Taplin
Peter & Dottie Telford
Graham & Maureen
  Thompson
Paul & Maureen Thompson
Jim & Lucy Tiflitis
Enzo & Pat Titaro
Vince & Carmel Tripodi

CONTENTS

INTRODUCTION

"The Primary cause of our disease is in us, always in us."
Antoine Beachamp 1883

"You have cancer". Three words that to many would conjure up images of defeat. I have heard these words, yet with the help and love of those whom I believe are put on this earth for the example they provide, I have declared war on this disease. I am fighting the enemy. I will never surrender.

It is my unshakeable belief that the contraction of cancer, or any other disease for that matter, is brought about by ourselves. If you believe that the cause of a disease is attributable to 'bad luck', an event beyond your control, then I'm afraid you have been misinformed. You must understand that basic tenet: it has been caused by ourselves. What I mean by 'ourselves' is our environment and the ways of our current society.

I do not wish to preach. The purpose of this book is rather to provide a practical guide to anyone with cancer or any other disease, to locate the necessary information and, once put into action, they can travel along the road to recovery as I have. It won't be easy. Nothing worthwhile ever is.

If you, or someone you know, has been diagnosed with cancer — or any other ailment for that matter — this book will help if you wish to keep your body and mind healthy and prevent any serious ailments. Within these pages, you will find practical tips and information that you can arm yourself with, which will allow you to engage with me in the battle against disease. I also hope that you will find a lot of love and discover that you are not alone.

It has been designed as a self-help source. In accordance with that principle, the groundwork has to be laid down by you, the reader.

The steps that I recommend you take before plunging forward are as follows:

1. Don't panic into believing that you will die tomorrow if you don't find a cure today. It is a known fact that fear can kill well before any disease has a chance to. Whenever I felt scared, I would pray and I wouldn't stop praying until I realised there was nothing to be scared of.

2. There are literally hundreds of types of cancer, however only a handful of these are aggressive, so don't be forced into undertaking immediate surgery, radiation or chemotherapy without first knowing the facts and the alternative options available.

3. Accept what you have and don't make a big deal of it. The reasons for this will become obvious. Get on with the task at

hand and treat it as if it were another nagging cold. Don't go looking for complex answers to a simple solution.

4. Above all, use your common sense. Don't be intimidated by your doctor. Ask questions, as simple as you think they may be.

5. Finally, let logic be your guide.

Along the way, a lot of my story with cancer will permeate through. It is my sincere desire that within my story, you will find inspiration, hope, a touch of humour and of course, LOVE.

The crux of the book is to provide you with an option. An option which will enable you to make your own decision as to the type of treatment you prefer to follow.

There clearly has to be a natural way. I fervently believe that there is. My family and I are living proof of this.

As you read on, you will find out about the Gerson treatment and other treatments, how to purify your drinking water, how to set up an enema and more to the point what IS an enema? Don't worry, I won't be blinding you with science or any of its jargon. I will be with you every step of the way explaining each and every issue as it arises.

You will hopefully grow to love and appreciate the inviolable rules of Nature, of which we are so much a part. We need to get back to Nature, to drink in its beauty and breathe in its life sustaining force.

The treatment which has strengthened my belief and sustained me is the previously mentioned Gerson Therapy. As you will discover, this scientifically validated treatment is a practical encapsulation of the Nature-as-a-cure principle.

May my book be a tribute to a man who swam against the current of mainstream thought and fought for what he believed in:

THE PRESERVATION OF LIFE.

THE TURNING POINT: MY 'NEW MIND' IS BORN

"Replace panic with prayer, fear with faith and overcome death itself".

Proverb

I was getting dressed to go out one evening and as I was pulling on my jeans, I experienced an excruciating pain in my left testicle. The pain was so severe, I was sent into shock.

Once the initial onslaught subsided, I made a decision. Whatever caused this pain, whatever caused this shock, would remain, for the time being at least, my secret. I even concealed the incident from my wife. Why worry her when the incident may just have been 'one of those things'! As you can probably guess, I was in a state of denial, trying my hardest to mentally block out the incident.

My mind, as you would expect, was a whirlwind. Denial on the one hand, determination to find out more on the other. Serving as an undercurrent was my refusal to disclose my condition to anyone. In hindsight, I can see that this need to go it alone suited my purpose well and can serve as a practical demonstration of what this book wishes to impart. Do you want to cure your condition? First and foremost, don't panic yourself, get down to your own resources, listen to your inner self and realise that you are surrounded by loved ones that truly want to help. Do not underestimate the healing power of your body, it has a natural healing ability.

Of course, you will need the support and assistance of others, but at least if you apply your mind and intelligently weigh up all the options, then you will engage in the battle on your own terms.

I realised just how negative society is towards cancer treatment when I viewed a television programme on the subject several years ago. A scientist, qualified up to his eyeballs, was telling all and sundry that in his professional opinion, cancer of the testicle was affecting more and more males. It was a very negative prognosis with the only 'breakthrough' being the scientist's belief that this form of cancer COULD be related to the wearing of tight pants. This was so vague as to be negligible.

I realised that if I took on board the opinion of mainstream medicine as it related to cancer, my battle would be severely compromised. This opinion is based on my personal observation of hundreds of cancer patients undergoing chemotherapy and radiotherapy. I realise that there was the potential to become demoralised and as any 'soldier' will tell you, demoralisation is one item NOT welcome.

The overall perspective of the programme was, I felt, symptomatic of society's peculiar 'need' to hear negativity.

Sociologists are of course more qualified to speak on this subject than I am, but as far as I am concerned, this 'willingness' by society to take on board negativity seems increasingly to be the case. I dislike this aspect of society. Moreover, I reject it.

The mindset of the doctor fortunately does not reflect the facts. According to several specialists and doctors I visited, the success rate of this type of cancer is close to 95%. The situation is therefore not as bleak as we have been led to believe.

I recently read an article in "Time" magazine relating to the rapid decline in male fertility *(Time magazine, 18 March 1996)*. In a comprehensive analysis covering 15,000 men from 21 countries, Danish scientists discovered an alarming fall of nearly 50% in average sperm counts in only the last 50 years. They reported that one of the possible causes for this decline in sperm count, was due to chemical pollutants in the environment. They finally added that if this rate of decline continues, the average male will be infertile within a century.

I needed to hold on to the positives of my situation lest I succumbed to the prevailing negative attitude towards cancer. In this endeavour, I was aided tremendously by the positive example of Marisa, my cousin, who had been diagnosed with breast cancer. For the time being of course, I couldn't share with her my situation. I still withheld the information from my loved ones and would continue to do so for several months.

That time period was certainly an experience. I researched, I consulted, but above all, I contemplated. My condition brought to the fore thoughts of my mortality. How, in the worse case scenario, my death would impact on those left behind. Yes, I would be lying to you if I said that thoughts of death did not enter my mind. Again, I was engaged in battle, the battle within my mind. The battle of the mind is the decisive one. Your success hinges on how strong you can make this vital asset.

Having said that, I need to assert that positive thinking, as with all things in Nature, does not exist in a vacuum. Practicalities of life need to be attended to.

CANCER CRUSADE

"To wish to be well is part of becoming well".

Seneca

While I was in a state of emotion, I decided to hit the road in what I refer to as my 'Mobile Crusade' in August 1995.

Using my work van, I embarked on a fund-raising drive for the Anti-Cancer Foundation. My motivation for this venture was two-fold. Firstly, it was a gesture on my part to contribute something worthwhile to society. I had no way of knowing just how long I had left in this world, so I decided that if my number was up, I needed to do something positive. Secondly, it was an effective way to raise funds and awareness in order to combat this disease.

Call it idealistic, call it dramatic, call it what you will, but it was something I felt I just had to do. Time was of the essence, as I felt the tumour was growing.

The bottom line was that I raised over A$20,000 by selling advertising space on my van to various businesses. Far and away from any other considerations however, was the satisfaction of setting an example for my children. Through this, I hoped that they witnessed their father returning something back to society.

Little did I know it then, but my campaign was to serve as the catalyst for the event that literally changed and saved my life.

The letter

I received a letter from an anonymous source. It arrived as a result of the publicity generated by my cancer drive. The letter informed me of various cancer therapies by different physicians, in particular one by Dr Max Gerson (1881-1959), a name that does not immediately spring to one's mind when discussing medical revolutionaries. Yet that is how I see him; a physician who flew in the face of mainstream wisdom as he strove to treat the cancer patients referred to him to the best of his ability.

John Cirocco
  John with his 'Cancer Crusader' vehicle

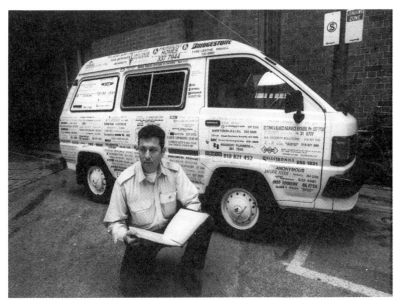

His best, I say without fear of contradiction, was certainly good enough.

Without delay, I purchased his book, "A CANCER THERAPY", (Fifth Edition, ©1990. Published by The Gerson Institute, Ed. Gar Hildenbrand). To say that I was affected by this book would be an understatement. I felt Dr Gerson's love for humanity emanating from every page as he wrote in a language easy to understand by anyone who sought his opinion.

Moreover, I had found a kindred spirit. As for the person who wrote that letter to me; if you are reading this book, all I can say to you is, "Thank you from my heart, you saved my life".

Following I would like to share with you the letter sent to me by my 'Angel':

Dear John,

I am writing to you because I can see that you are a man with a big heart. Your fund-raising efforts are admirable but I regret to inform you that you are directing money to the wrong place.

The fact is that cancer is not the terror that doctors want people to feel, it is curable and has been for decades. Chemotherapy, radiotherapy and disfiguring surgery, are not the answer.

They are painful, dehumanising and they flatten the morale which in turn flattens the immune system. They do more harm than good but these three procedures are making millions of dollars for drug companies, machinery manufacturers, doctors, surgeons, hospitals and pathology services. The latter are springing up all over the place, why?

I am sending you some information which hopefully will show you what I mean.

Have you heard of Essiac? It is a cure for cancer made up of four common herbs. It has cured cancer for decades, but the cancer industry has gone to extraordinary lengths to suppress the knowledge of it. Early this year, the Australian Therapeutic Goods Administration closed down the importers of the product, based in Perth. The four herbs in Essiac are harmless, have no side effects and work! I know a woman who was sent home to die of breast cancer, and who has been able to arrest the disease using nutrition and Essiac. Why do doctors send people home to die of cancer, when referring them to herbal remedies can save their lives?! It is because greed comes first.

I don't blame you if you are shocked by this information. I was too. I wish you all the best.

"A person who hates to see good people conned".

The letter also contained copies of literature extracted from various journals relating to different therapies and as I mentioned before, in particular, Dr Max Gerson's Therapy.

As you can imagine, my first reaction to this letter was one of horror, followed by intense anger and I nearly threw the letter in the bin. But questions started entering my mind. Would the medical profession really suppress a natural cancer therapy coming onto the market? Surely if there were a cure for cancer, researchers would have told us about it, wouldn't they?

The first step

I may not have been able to consult with Dr Gerson personally — more's the pity — but I could avail myself of his legacy.
Summoning my courage, I telephoned Dr Gerson's daughter Charlotte in Bonita, California, (The Gerson Institute, PO Box 430, Bonita CA 92002 USA. Tel: (619) 267 1150) and instantly was struck by the fact that the love I had felt in Dr Gerson's writing was also evident in his daughter. I felt his spirit.

Her advice to me was to get a diagnosis, undergo a C.T. scan and then go to Mexico, where the Gerson Institute is based. She made it all sound so simple. For me, it was all a tremendously emotional experience, yet I still could not share the full details with anyone at the time.

This is a trait of mine, one which my General Practitioner mildly scolded me for when I finally consulted him. Having not done anything about my condition for several months, I only went to see him after being urged by Anna because I told her I felt a little run down. She advised me to go directly one Saturday morning before starting work. Upon examining me, he took action immediately. I undertook a C.T. scan the same day.

What did surprise me, was my composure during these proceedings. I didn't faint, become morose or angry. In actual fact, I was very calm and focused. I can only attribute this to the new found strength that I had gleaned from Charlotte Gerson, an extension of her father.

The C.T. scan discovered the disconcerting fact that there was a spot in my right lung and that several lymph nodes in my groin were inflamed. Despite this, the positive feeling that I alluded to earlier, once again came into play. Moreover, I felt that a new journey had begun. The amazing thing was that I could access latent reservoirs of strength from which I could draw on. This strength gave me focus. I had a task ahead of me and I was not prepared to shy away from it.

The next step was to inform Anna. It was at this point that I fully realised just how important she is to me. She became my Rock of Gibraltar, a person I could rely on wholeheartedly and without reservation. The story of my battle with cancer is also Anna's.

Having said that, it remains to be said that Anna's initial reaction to the news was to have been expected under the circumstances. As is my habit, I kicked it off by saying, "We're going to America!" in a flippant manner. With that introduction I attempted to impart the rest of the details in as calm a manner as possible. For all that, Anna was at first incredulous and then came the shock, the tears, the over-riding sense of denial. It was nevertheless, an incredibly bonding experience between us, one which would carry us through the trying events that were to follow. I was the pilot and Anna was my navigator. Marshalling our combined strengths, we declared war on cancer.

Over that weekend, it was incredible to watch the reactions of our respective families when the news broke. Tears flowed, shock set in and the common phrase "Why you?" came into play. After assuring them of my plans, the overall reaction was positive, no doubt this was due to the fact that Anna and I dealt with it in a positive manner.

I do recall one house party that Anna hosted just before we left (I refused to let her cancel it) some people froze uncertain of how to react, but generally, the reaction was very positive. In fact, we received around one hundred telephone calls in support. I developed partial laryngitis answering them all!

An interesting weekend, to say the least!

On Monday 25 September 1995, I had an appointment with my first surgeon. Upon examining me and referring to the blood test, he confirmed the lump to be cancerous and that judging by the swollen appearance of my lymph nodes in the area of my groin, there may possibly be some spread. His recommendations were:

a) remove the affected testicle via a small incision in the scrotum
b) remove all swollen lymph nodes in the groin and along the thorax area of the body (that is the centre line of the body)
c) commence with regional radiation therapy to kill any cancer cells still around, and
d) a required dose of chemotherapy just to be sure.

He also asked if I had any children, as the radiation would damage the remaining testicle, causing me to be sterile.

He told me the operation would be a quick and simple one, with a minimum stay in hospital and that the success rate for this type of cancer was between 90-95%. He then insisted I have the operation the following morning. However, what he did fail to tell me was that if the spot in the right lung was also cancerous, my prognosis would not be as promising. Needless to say, I didn't have the operation the next day.

On Tuesday, my GP recommended I see a competent chemotherapy specialist which I reluctantly did. He was my first taste of how intimidating this profession can be. Maybe it was because I was asking him too many questions of which he did not feel comfortable, or maybe because of the negativity I showed toward his toxic drugs.

On Wednesday, buoyed by an incredible outpouring of support from friends and family, Anna and I immediately started making plans and preparations to travel overseas on the next leg of our journey, Mexico and the Gerson Institute.

Our tickets and visas were organised within the space of a few days, such was the urgency of our quest. We were aided a great deal by the contribution of a substantial amount of money provided unconditionally by our families. This was an incredible act of faith on their part and one which Anna and I will always be grateful for.

It wasn't all plain sailing, of course. We encountered bureaucratic red tape — or should that be, sheer bloody mindedness — in the shape of a clerk at the Australian Consulate in Melbourne. He was reluctant to issue our visas as, in his opinion, a cure for cancer could be found in Australia. We of course begged to differ, but in order to get to Mexico as soon as possible, we had no choice but to pay the 'necessary' collateral in order to smooth our passage. Having dealt with this impediment, we were on our way. You see, the government doesn't want charity cases. I had to show them that I had the money to undertake the therapy. More than was necessary.

Leaving our beloved children Olivia and Christian behind was the hardest thing we have ever had to do. Under the circumstances, this trip was not one which we could take them on.

Arriving in Los Angeles, on Friday 29 September 1995, we caught a charter flight to San Diego, from where we were picked up by a Hospital transport mini bus and taken to Tijuana, Mexico. Many details flew by me in a flurry. I didn't take everything in, as I was too wrapped up in the task at hand. Anna bought herself a travel journal before we left and filled in the details, from when I told her the news to when we left Mexico to come home.

When reading her journal at a later stage, the memories came flooding back, the trip to the hospital, the environment, the people, the atmosphere.

Before being picked up by the transit bus to take us to the Gerson Clinic, we had spent an extra hour in the San Diego Airport because we had missed our connecting flight from LA Airport. Unlike our Adelaide Airport, the LA Airport resembles the size of our city. By the time we passed through customs, found transit buses to take us to the appropriate terminals and locate the correct flight counter, we missed our flight. Luckily another would be leaving within the hour. I must say, when we finally did board, we felt we boarded a toy plane. We had never travelled on a charter plane before, so to say we felt a little nervous, is an understatement!

The flight was only 30 minutes and to our surprise, it wasn't at all bad. With a little prayer and high hopes, we landed safely in San Diego Airport. We managed to contact the Gerson Clinic to notify them of our delay, and luckily the driver was to make a final pick-up for the day — US!

The drive to the Mexican border was pleasant but as mentioned before, my mind was in a whirlwind. I do recall though, the sight at the Mexican border. Cars were lined up for miles, on both sides! Being from the Gerson Clinic, the driver was allowed clearance in a special lane with no hold up, due to the frequent trips made during the course of one day. These long queues are imperative to stop drug trafficking and illegitimate foreigners crossing the border.

Many Mexican citizens have special permits which allow them to cross the border every day to work in the United States. For these Mexicans, this is a Godsend, as the pay in the States is considerably more than in Mexico, and the dollar is worth a lot more, so they have a comfortable lifestyle in Mexico although it means early starts and late returns each day.

Generally, Mexico is a very poor country, and this is apparent soon after crossing the border. Scattered all over land in the mountains, are shanties. These small homes are made of cardboard and any other scraps of materials found, to construct these homes. They have no running water, electricity or modern commodities. The people living in these homes are known as squatters, as they construct their homes on land belonging to the government, in exchange for welfare. It made us realise, how fortunate we are and for the little luxuries we have.

Driving into Tijuana felt good, I knew we were nearing our destination. Tijuana, what I saw of it, which was very little, seemed to be a modest city. Anna would go walking almost every day, and she noticed that there were portions of streets with neat tidy houses, and sections with very old run down homes. Overall it was pleasant.

It was a peculiar feeling to say the least to arrive and enter the Gerson Clinic. The place that I had read about came alive, took shape for me as I stood there soaking in the atmosphere. The culture shock was all pervading. I had visions of it being Third World in appearance, yet here we were, in a highly professional, well maintained centre, dedicated to the eradication of disease.

Most of the staff spoke broken English, with the exception of the doctors. However, we got by. I was too keen to start my therapy to let language impede on my task!

Assigned to our room, Anna and I found that we couldn't unpack. So much was riding on this, raised hopes, wariness of the unknown. All we could do was to be patient, trust our instincts and the professionals at the Clinic, and see this through.

MEXICO

The therapy begins

There was no time to let wavering thoughts bog me down, however justified they may have been. I sat in on a lecture that very afternoon we arrived and it was there, in that room, that my head was re-attuned, I regained my focus. The clinic held lectures Monday to Friday which ran for approximately three

Max Gerson Memorial Cancer Centre
Tel: 0011-1880-759-2966 Email: compuserve 75141.2044@gerson.org
Web page: http//www/1999.com/gerson/

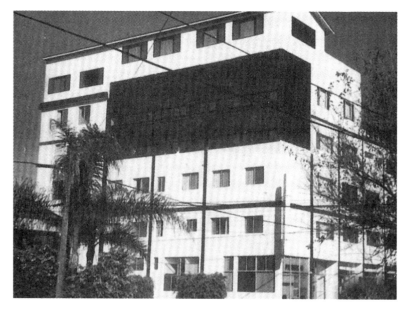

hours. I attended and taped every one. The lectures were given by doctors, oncologists, epidemiologists and Charlotte Gerson.

The lectures would vary from cooking lessons to preparing and administering injections to medical lectures. It was at these lectures that you could say I was thrown in the deep end of alternative medicine. I was introduced to therapies such as Laetrile (B17), CoQ10, Hydrogen Peroxide, Ozone, Essiac, shark cartilage, H.B.O., multi-vitamin therapy, Hyperthermia, etc.

To say I was confused, would be an understatement. My thirst for alternative knowledge helped me learn more about these therapies. They also spoke on subjects such as water purification, natural forms of pain relief, dental amalgams and certain aspects of our environment in general.

From the onset, one thing was made quite clear. Before any of the above therapies can start, the issue of nutrition must be addressed. The Gerson therapy took care of this totally. This was reinforced when Anna gave me my first carrot juice.

When I left our room to attend the lecture, Anna remained to catch up on some rest. Unfortunately as she recalls, it wasn't long before a knock at the door brought her to her feet. She opened the door and who she presumed to be a nurse was pointing to her feet and saying "shoes" or so Anna thought. She remembers feeling angry that she couldn't even walk around barefoot in our own room. It was only after the nurse turned out to be a kitchen hand, that Anna realised that what she was saying was "juice" not "shoes". That is where broken English was a real challenge. Little comments like this make me smile and remember all the warm and loving friends we made in Mexico. We met people from all walks of life. Many were Americans, then there were Canadians, Asians, Germans, English and Italians to mention a few. The following are some of the people we met. Karl and Marnae from Washington DC, Tom and Johanna from California, Diane and Jenny from Georgia, Atlanta, Annie and Carole from England, Fabiola and Flora from Italy, Alois and Margaret from Germany, Don and Gary from Houston, Texas, Miki from New York, Claude and Mary from Arizona, Nathan and Joy from Texas, Martin and Victoria from Germany, Creed, Kathleen and Gina from Ohio, and Richard and Vivien from Canada. We met many other people but did not get the chance to know them well, as the ones already mentioned. Most of the patients were being treated for cancer, however, there were a number of patients with varying ailments, from strokes to Hepatitis C, and even heroin addiction. Many of the patients we met, came from professional backgrounds ie. doctors, surgeons, lawyers etc. Although complete strangers at first, we all formed a bond that most do not achieve in a life time. Not a day goes by that both Anna and myself do not think of these wonderful people.

The general atmosphere of the clinic was serene. The rooms were very modest in appearance and each had its own ensuite. Because of sewerage problems, toilet paper could not be flushed, but was placed into waste paper baskets instead, which would be emptied out by cleaners every day. They would also

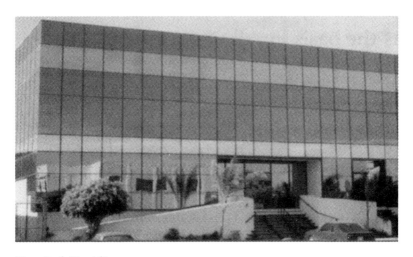

Hospital Meridian
   Tel: 0011-619-585-7600 Fax: 0011-585-7610.
   Web page: http//www.gerson.org Email: info@gerson.org

bring fresh towels and supplies as requested. There was no airconditioning in the rooms except for the dining, lounge and lecture areas. Fortunately at the time we were there, in October, the weather was mild every day as it was their autumn.

For the patients like myself, whose general health was good, the days would be spent relaxing, sitting in on lectures and chatting amongst ourselves. There were no televisions in our individual rooms, so any viewing would be done as a group, normally after dinner. There was a lovely upstairs balcony/patio area with sunchairs and umbrellas to enjoy. The days flew by very quickly, as every hour something needed to be administered, swallowed or eaten. At the beginning of our stay, I was on a high and would go from room to room chatting with patients and their companions, encouraging and sharing our mutual fears and hopes. But, as I got deeper into the therapy, I found I needed to rest more so that the therapy could have the full effect.

Several weeks after returning home, we were notified that the Gerson Clinic had relocated to Hospital Meridien DePlayas De Tijuana.

A TYPICAL GERSON ROUTINE

6.00 am   Rise and shine for your first coffee enema (which were soon to be known as 'Coffee Breaks') of the day.

7.00 am   Liver and Vitamin B12 injection and vitals taken (ie. blood pressure and temperature).

7.30 am   3 Wobe Mugos (digestive enzymes) taken with water *(see Medication Table, page 241)*.

8.00 am   *Breakfast*

First juice of day, one glass of orange juice taken with medication: 2 Acidol Pepsin, 1 Thyroid, 1 Niacin, 3 Pancreatin *(see Medication Table, page 241)*.

Bowl of oatmeal in porridge form served with stewed fruits and honey.

Fresh fruit and special home baked raisin bread.

9.00 am   Carrot juice

9.30 am   Green juice (apple, capsicum, green leaves.) *(see The Therapy for proportions, page 84)*.

10.00 am   Carrot & apple juice (1 Thyroid, 1 Niacin, 2 CoQ10)

Coffee enema

Plate of fresh fruit

11.00 am   Carrot juice (2 Liver capsules)

12.00 pm   Green juice

12.30 pm   3 Wobe mugos

1.00 pm   ***Lunch***

Carrot juice (2 acidol pepsin, 1 thyroid, 1 niacin, 3 pancreatin, 2 CoQ10)

Bowl of Hippocrates soup *(see Food, page 178)*

Baked potato in jacket

Green salad (organic red wine vinegar diluted with water, served as dressing)

Variety of vegetables, baked or boiled

Fresh fruit

2.00 pm   Green juice

Coffee enema

3.00 pm   Carrot juice (2 liver capsules)

Fresh fruit platter.

4.00 pm   Carrot & apple juice (2 Liver Capsules)

5.00 pm   Carrot & apple juice (1 thyroid, 1 niacin, 3 pancreatin, 3 wobe mugos)

6.00 pm   Green juice (1 niacin, 2 CoQ10)

6.30 pm   3 Wobe Mugos

7.00 pm   ***Dinner***

Carrot juice (2 acidol pepsin, 1 thyroid, 1 niacin, 3 pancreatin)

Hippocrates soup

Baked potato

Salad, Variety of vegetables

Fresh fruit

10.00 pm   Last coffee enema of day.

Patients on the full Gerson Therapy, meaning patients who had not previously undergone chemotherapy, were given castor oil every second day with their enemas. Rise and shine at 5.00 am for 1 tablespoon of castor oil by mouth followed by cup of black coffee then back to bed. The second tablespoon of castor oil is used in the 10.00 am enema with the difference that it is released as soon as it is instilled. *(Preparation advice given in page 108)*.

Not exactly a 'fun' regime, the full impact of this did not sink in until lights out at 11.00 pm every night. It was during these quiet times that I reflected on the treatment, the ramifications and any thoughts that I may have had. I never bucked the system. I simply went with the flow, knowing that I had little choice to do otherwise. If little nagging thoughts began to creep in during these reflective moments, they were increasingly repelled by the series of what I call weird and wonderful things that were beginning to happen.

PHYSICAL SIDE EFFECTS

Eczema: I had been plagued by this skin disorder since I was nineteen. After the first week of therapy, the eczema on my face cleared up; the eczema on my scalp went the same way on the second week, as simple as that. This was the first tangible evidence that the therapy was working.

Lipoma cysts: These benign, fatty cysts, had been steadily growing over the last five years on my legs. After a couple of weeks of the therapy, they had reduced in size. This also was a most welcome side effect.

Eye irritation: The red and yellow irritation around my pupils began to clear up after one week.

Body odour: Pre-therapy, this had been somewhat of an embarrassment to me, requiring liberal doses of deodorants. Not any more, all I now require is a mild soap. No doubt the therapy was eradicating the toxins from my body.

Weight: Due to the intensive diet and detoxification, I lost 9kg in the space of three weeks, my metabolism improved.

These side effects, (as welcoming as they were), were of course peripheral to the main objective.

It was with great relief that after just one week of therapy, I noticed that the inflammation in my groin area had decreased. ONE WEEK!

If any doubts filtered through my head, these were counteracted by these more than welcome developments. They reinforced in my mind the conviction that the Gerson Therapy is a life saving therapy. A therapy which bypasses the need for what we would call mainstream or orthodox methods, such as radiation and chemotherapy.

Although at first glance the therapy may seem a little overwhelming, consider the situation if you are in a life threatening position. Do you go through months of experiencing, or watching a loved one experience, pain, loss of appetite, loss of hair, physical and emotional changes with no guarantees from chemotherapy or radiation, or do you discipline and re-organise your lifestyle to adapt to a healthier diet and lifestyle? As brushing your teeth is a routine and a part of everyday living, so is the Gerson Therapy.

By the time you are ready to set upon your journey to better health, a better life, you will be able to re-organise your kitchen and habits with a minimum of fuss.

From being stressed out and overworked with my business, unfit and unhealthy to say the least, I've come through a strict regime to a maintenance diet, and more importantly, I now have a closeness and love for my wife and children that many may not have the time in their busy schedules to enjoy thoroughly.

Throughout the last two years, I have learnt to live my life as if each day is my last!

The major component of the Gerson Therapy is centred around high-grade organic foods, including a variety of juices, Hippocrates soup *(see Food Recipes, page 178)*, and organic fruit and vegetables.

I became a vegetarian overnight! I had but two choices; take it or leave it. Initially, I favoured the latter, as I was not impressed with the monotony of my meals, but of course my taste buds eventually became more receptive as the worth of the diet was made clear to me.

FAMILY MEDICAL HISTORY

"Nature will never follow people, but people will have to follow the laws of nature."

Discorides (AD40-90)

The Gerson Therapy once applied to my family, had benefits that I can only describe as miraculous. It is essential to detail such developments, because it proves that the therapy is all embracing and is not limited to the treatment of cancer alone. In fact, upon reading "A CANCER THERAPY", by Max Gerson, you will discover that he stumbled upon the therapy for cancer when he originally applied the treatment to cure his life long migraines.

This is of course a benefit of the therapy that I am pleased to detail, as you can appreciate, the health of my family is of paramount importance to me.

Anna

MIGRAINES

I recall that during our courting days Anna experienced frequent headaches and migraines as well as significant pain in her neck. The pain became so severe that bed rest was often called for. It was a mystery ailment, the cause of which escaped us. Was it derived from her puberty or the long term effects of the car accident Anna was involved in years before?

Whatever the origin, we took action and before too long, Anna was being bombarded with a wide range of medication.

When the pain became severe, Anna was subjected to injections. The upshot of all this treatment was that Anna's condition actually worsened, and by September 1993, her neck aches and migraines were so severe that they became unbearable. A C.T. scan was performed and the diagnosis gave Anna the 'all clear'. Her consultations with her chiropractor only offered mild relief, the mystery deepened.

CHRONIC FATIGUE (EPSTEIN BARR VIRUS)

In December 1994, Anna kept complaining she was feeling very tired and run down but pushed it aside as we all tend to do.

During the following months, Anna kept complaining of fatigue and in July 1995 she was finally diagnosed as suffering from Chronic Fatigue Syndrome. After several blood tests, she was told that she had the glandular fever virus in her system for several months, it was no longer present but ultimately had triggered the chronic fatigue.

Her course of action consisted of monthly injections of B12 and Alertonic, a syrup to give her extra energy. These treatments had questionable worth, although the B12 shots helped a little. Overall however, her physical and mental states were low to say the least.

She was constantly tired, run down and miserable. A simple task such as preparing breakfast for the children would bring her to tears as she felt it was such an effort to do. She would literally get up from bed in the morning, straight to the sofa to sleep again, and that was after she had been sleeping from 7.30 pm the previous night! Anna of course tried to help herself, but exhaustion invariably took over. Sleep offered no respite.

This was all before Anna tried the MODIFIED Gerson Therapy. Once she became adept, the results were almost immediate. These became apparent after less than one week on the treatment! It also needs to be stressed here that she placed herself on a reduced regime consuming three juices a day, and one coffee enema.

She started to regain more energy and her head and neck aches disappeared. As simple as that. Also at this point I would like to mention that Anna was a true chocaholic. She would consume chocolate almost every day. Being on the therapy in Mexico, even partners of patients would have the same menu and it was there we noticed that all her pain disappeared. They definitely did not have chocolate treats! She has for the most part, stayed clear of chocolates knowing that they will bring on a headache instantly. This is fact, as on several occasions she could not resist the temptation of her favourite treat so she indulged. The result, instant headache!

Furthermore, after having lived on medication for most of her early teens and adult life, she has no medication for pain. When there has been pain due to her indulgence, a Triad *(see pages 122, 241)* and a quick enema rectified the problem.

Another ailment that soon disappeared was Anna's pins and needles in her arms that started when she was pregnant with our twins. The pain was at its highest threshold when she was in her second trimester and continued to the end of her pregnancy. The pain diminished somewhat after the birth of the twins but continued in a mild form for the next four years.

To see your loved one lifted of such burdens right before your very eyes, is truly a heart-warming experience, I can assure you.

As I watched her progress, I realised that I was witnessing a miracle in action. Even her eyesight improved as a result of the therapy.

It was upon returning from Mexico and engrossing myself in a variety of literature and medical books that I consulted "The Australian Drug Guide" (Third Edition, ©1995, by Dr Jonathan Upthal). I highly recommend this very informative source, detailing as it does, information on an extensive range of medications — their constituents, effectiveness and all other relevant information. There is even a pronunciation guide for the lay person.

My upbeat assessment of the book aside, it actually raised more questions than it answered. One in particular concerned an Aspirin like medication, but more potent. It is prescribed for the control of pain and the reversal of swelling and stiffness of inflamed joints, the objective being the improvement of mobility. Consulting "The Australian Drug Guide" I discovered that this drug is known to have bad effects on cartilage repair, often causing rapid joint deterioration. This raises the all too pertinent question: why was this drug recommended to Anna, when its effects directly contradicted every thing we were trying to do? Although it alleviated Anna's pain slightly, the underlying 'benefit' of the drug was that it was damaging her cartilage!

What also needed to be made redundant was our diet. Junk food, that dead, frozen, non-combustible food, loved unfortunately by millions, was assigned to the circular file (ie. 'the bin'), to be replaced with the organic variety. Spring water became our favoured beverage.

MODIFIED GERSON THERAPY

The following is the modified version of the Gerson Therapy which Anna undertook in Mexico and continued for the next three months at home, which not only rid her of migraines and Chronic Fatigue, but ultimately corrected the problems which had previously inhibited her natural ability to conceive.

Morning

1 glass carrot or mixed vegetable juice (*see Juices, page 118*)

1 bowl of porridge with stewed fruits

1 banana (optional — can be sliced in porridge)

1 piece fruit toast with scrape of butter (Wuppertaler Rye Fruit Loaf is the one we eat as it is both wheat and yeast free. (Made in Victoria. Available in selected health shops nationally).

Mid morning

Fresh fruit

Lunch

1 glass carrot juice

1 baked potato

1 bowl vegetable soup (*Hippocrates, see Food, page 178*)

Salad

Combination steamed vegetables

Mid afternoon

Fresh fruit

Dinner

Same as lunch, with vegetables and salads differing in variety and combinations.

Additionally

Also 1-2 litres of spring water consumed throughout the day.

Anna undertook the above modified therapy strictly for four weeks, then once we returned home she slowly added a little brown rice, plain yoghurt, quark (available at health stores), deep sea fish and chicken to her diet. The fish and chicken was always grilled or poached and kept to once a week.

Whilst on this programme, Anna would have one coffee enema every day at around 9 pm. She found this schedule very uplifting and invigorating. As a support to this programme she would take various supplements with each meal. These consisted of:

1 digestive enzyme before every meal
1 1000mg tablet of Vitamin C after every meal
1 50mg niacin with meals
1 multivitamin capsule taken with breakfast only

All supplements are available from health stores or naturopaths.

TEAS

Some teas which were and still are of great benefit are:

Camomile & peppermint   *– Digestion*
Red clover blossom   *– PMT*
Red clover with stinging nettle   *– Blood purification and toning*
Dandelion root   *– Liver detox*

There are many other teas available for various ailments and these are all available from health stores. A good reference guide to herbs is "Healing through God's Pharmacy" by Maria Treben (ISBN 3-85068-124-6).

At this point I would like to mention that whilst on this programme, Anna continued to make thirteen juices a day for me, prepare three meals, five enemas, shopping, general house duties, organise the twins, and still have time to do gardening in between for her own pleasure (May I also add, she was four months pregnant at the time). This may seem like an unbelievable achievement, which Anna now admits she still doesn't know how she did it, but what she puts it down to, is organisation, dedication and love.

No change of life is easy and our adoption of the Gerson Therapy and all it entailed was no exception. Throwing away the habits of a lifetime was no easy task, but we persevered, confident that we simply had no other alternative. We had tried mainstream methods and they had failed us. There clearly had to be another way. We were on a steep learning curve, but the journey was worthwhile if our family was to go forward, unencumbered by the milestone of ill health. It was time to apply the therapy to our children — THE FUTURE.

OUR CHILDREN

"Patience is the essence of the soul."

Proverb

Christian

CHRONIC ASTHMA

The health of our son Christian has always been of major concern to Anna and myself. Up until the age of twelve months he had been a healthy baby and his progress was quite satisfactory. Sadly, this all changed when he entered his second year. Bouts of persistent, unproductive coughing were commonplace, an alarming development I can assure you. Ironically, we had never specifically taken him to be examined for this. It was upon a routine paediatrician visit that the subject was first raised. After examination, Anna was asked about his general health. Anna confirmed that she was happy with his progress except for the constant nagging cough Christian was having. After establishing a pattern of coughing periods, the diagnosis was Chronic Asthma.

Acting immediately, we administered a preventative drug commonly prescribed for this condition, via a nebuliser pump therapy kit, three times a day until the coughing stabilised. This routine was to continue for several months and a record kept until the next visit. If a further attack occurred, a more powerful drug would be prescribed, again via the nebuliser. The bottom line was that despite our best intentions, after two years on this medication, Christian's condition did not improve. The coughing attacks continued unabated.

What also was of great concern to us were the other ailments that plagued Christian.

He was constantly tired and his concentration levels were low. Frustrated, he often erupted into bouts of screaming. Some side effects of the medication made Christian hyperactive and he lost his appetite. It was a constant struggle trying to keep him nourished and hydrated. As if all this wasn't enough for such a young person, Christian would suffer from severe constipation. Laxatives were administered and if the condition became unbearable, a glycerine suppository was given. Trips to the Children's Hospital were also necessary for this particular problem. As you can imagine, it was a heart wrenching time for us watching our little boy suffer from all this. No matter how big or small an ailment is in a child, I am sure all parents hate seeing their children suffer.

Christian became very upset for a week after his suppository, a very heart wrenching experience for us and painful for him. All we could do was try to help, to alleviate his suffering, to feel his pain.

We simply did not know any better. We administered this treatment because at the time we did not know of any other option. People would say to us that Christian would 'grow out of his asthma' but we were not so sure of the wisdom of that statement. We watched, we waited, we hoped.

I guess what we were waiting for was a miracle. That miracle came about for Christian via the Gerson Therapy just as surely as it did for Anna and myself. This of course is not to say that getting Christian on the diet was an easy task. Far from it. For a child that had been accustomed to junk food, the transformation to a healthy diet required a gradual process of painful acclimatisation. Needless to say, Christian was NOT a willing participant!

Gradually, we weaned him off his previous diet, which consisted mainly of milk (he loved it) and processed cheese. We gave him soya products, baked potatoes and of course, lots of organic fruits and vegetables, nuts and dried fruits. Sounds simple, doesn't it? Well, I can assure you that once Christian had become accustomed to the new regime, the results were almost immediate and heart-warming.

It is my pleasure to report that after one week on the diet, Christian's coughing attacks ceased. As simple as that. We realised that our earlier treatment of our son was tragically flawed, as we simply knew no better. We will never revert to our past practices.

Certain individuals asserted that Christian's condition improved because he simply 'grew out of it', but we know better. The results told us that the improvements that were becoming evident in Christian were of far reaching significance, too significant in fact to be attributable to merely 'growing out of it'. This latter prognosis is so vague as to be superfluous.

Consider the following: Christian's constipation has now been eliminated, his energy level has increased dramatically so that now he no longer requires mid-day naps as he did in the past and his lung capacity has also dramatically increased. The enlargement of his tonsils and adenoids which have always caused him to snore and reduce his oxygen intake, have returned to normal, nor is he required to have surgery to remove his tonsils as had been previously suggested.

Generally, he is now a stronger child. His quality of life has improved to such a level that we could not even dare to dream about such a development before adopting the Gerson Therapy.

I look forward to that day in the future when I can show Christian the box of medication he once had prescribed and tell him how we hoped in vain that they would help him.

Olivia

Our beloved daughter Olivia has also benefited from the Gerson Therapy. Her health was never as great a concern to us as her twin brother Christian, although she did contract the bronchiolitis virus as a young baby which fortunately dissipated. Olivia's needs were not as great as Christian's, so her adoption of the diet which incidentally, she took to with a

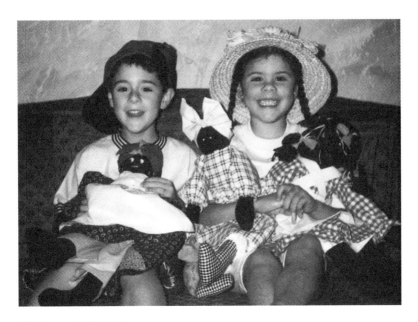

Olivia and Christian

minimum of fuss, can be seen as insurance for her future, rather than a remedy for any present illness.

As you would expect, our adoption of the Gerson Therapy created quite a few waves within our respective families. The therapy was so new to us all, naturally fear of the unknown made people wary and critical. Of course Anna and I had no guarantee that the therapy would work before tangible results could be witnessed. All we could do in the early days was plough through. We simply had to maintain our focus: we had absolutely no time for idle chit-chat. We had a job to do and that was to preserve the health of our family unit.

Not surprisingly perhaps, we became isolated, with people viewing us as if we were from another planet, spouting off about

our new life style. We were on a very steep learning curve —
we are STILL learning — and we know we simply could not
give up. We had to barge through the criticisms, the monotony
of the regime, if we were to give the therapy any real chance
of success.

I believe with all my heart, this experience has served as a
major bonding agent within our family. I am proud of what we
have achieved in the face of seemingly insurmountable
difficulties. It may seem an ironic, even peculiar thing to say,
but cancer changed my whole family for the better after we
adopted the Gerson way of life. We feel complete now, whole.
We feel, well … just great!

MY PERSONAL DEVELOPMENT

"Life has meaning only in the struggle. Triumph or defeat is in the hands of God, so let us celebrate the struggle."
Warrior Song

In the previous chapters, I have detailed the benefits that the Gerson Therapy had and is continuing to have on my family. At this point, I would like to describe my own personal development since returning from Mexico.

Shortly after arriving home, I noticed that my tumour had actually grown, but had softened quite a bit. This had become apparent in Mexico.

The cure was not instantly apparent. However, there were other positive benefits to come out of my journey and what follows is a blow-by-blow account of my progress.

FIRST WEEK BACK HOME

I underwent an operation to have my left testicle removed (Orchidectomy). This was a somewhat controversial decision on my behalf, but after weighing up my options I decided that removing the primary tumour would give my immune system a better fighting chance to clean up any lingering cancer cells. This procedure was simple and straightforward. My stay in hospital was minimal, three days.

In the three days I spent convalescing in hospital, Anna made several trips each day, bringing me fresh juices, enemas and food. She was there at 8.00 am in the morning with hot oatmeal and juice, then back at lunch and dinner. Upon being discharged I felt much stronger and was pleased to be going home to my family and my thirteen juices, eager to resume my lifesaving regime. Although my primary tumour had been removed I still needed to continue my therapy because I still did not want to receive chemotherapy or radiation which had been suggested to me.

By day six I was feeling a lot stronger especially after cleansing my body of the toxic drugs from the operation, via the coffee enemas. Being on the therapy prior to any operation is very good indeed because it makes your immune system a lot stronger and it can deal with drugs a lot better. Our bodies are very good to us and very strong indeed. Learn to respect it, and it will respect you. Exactly one week after the operation, I had an appointment with my surgeon. He was pleased with my progress, noting that there was no swelling and my drainage was very good from the incision. At this point, I told him about the Gerson Therapy. Not surprisingly, this was all new to him but instead of debunking it as I had been half expecting, he encouraged me to keep it up, as it obviously worked. This single positive comment, made me realise that there are orthodox practitioners out there, that would like to know more about the positive healing benefits of nutrition and alternative therapies. What I did tell him was that the prescribed next step to undergo chemotherapy and radiation was definitively NOT on my agenda. Thanks but definitively NO THANKS!

One person I was inspired by at this point was Dr Lorraine Day. An internationally acclaimed orthopedic surgeon, who was for fifteen years on the Faculty of the University of California San Francisco School of Medicine as Associate Professor and Vice Chairman of the Department of Orthopedics. She was also Chief of Orthopedic Surgery at San Francisco General Hospital and is recognised world-wide as an AIDS expert. She contracted breast cancer and defeated it. Her weapon? You guessed it — The Gerson Therapy.

I was amazed that someone like Dr Day, who practised orthodox medicine all her professional life, would become an advocate for alternative medicine. She expanded her field of references to include works on 'unorthodox' treatments and came away with the conviction that the Gerson Therapy together with other alternative therapies was the way to go. This information is available to us all. We just need to access the source. *(See Book Reviews, page 209)*.

Basically what I am saying is that it is essential for cancer patients to broaden their minds and field of reference so that they can, like Dr Day, myself, and thousands of others, equip ourselves with alternatives, judge the relative merits of the options put before them, and once having made an informed decision, go forward with the treatment that best suits their condition.

Many mainstream physicians are only conversant with 'procedure'. They use the tactic of thrusting upon the cancer patient a sense of urgency in order for him/her to act quickly. This misses one fundamental point about the contraction of cancer, and that is, the disease can take a long time to develop. Each case has to be judged on its own.

The majority of cancers are slow growing and before the symptoms appear, it may take up to ten or twenty years. Therefore I am baffled by this sense of urgency. Patients are not informed of any alternative treatments available. The diet is never addressed, yet diet is the ESSENTIAL factor as everything that we put into our bodies affects us in one way or another. With the information on the various therapies available and their relative merits, the individual can then make an informed decision —

IT'S YOUR LIFE

THE BALANCE SHEET

The approximate cost of undertaking the Gerson Therapy for almost four weeks including Anna was US$25,000. This figure included airfares for both myself and Anna, accommodation for four weeks in the Gerson Clinic, and medication for six months.

Optional costs include a Norwalk juicer ($4,000) and a water distiller ($4,000). Used Norwalk Juicers are available through cancer support groups in Australia. *(For new juicers, see page 109)*. As for water distillers, I have discovered it is much more economical to have distilled water delivered in 10L up to 20L containers. Once the patient has made him or herself conversant with the Gerson Therapy, they then come face to face with the old issue — finance. I bemoan the expenses that are incurred when undertaking the treatment and I count myself extremely fortunate that I had the family support, which enabled me to undertake the therapy. It is sad that health funds do not recognise this natural life saving therapy.

At this point, I would like to pass on some valuable information. If you intend to go to Mexico for the therapy as we did, then I suggest you ring around for a private health benefits fund that covers this type of therapy.

We did not know at the time that some health funds do not

cover alternative therapies, and although the Gerson Therapy is one of the few scientifically recognised therapies, we were refused any refund from our health fund. Another interesting discovery whilst talking to some of our fellow Gerson patients, was that many of the health funds in Germany recognise alternative therapies and some funds even give individuals discounts if they don't smoke or drink alcohol and if they meditate on a daily basis.

Undertaking the therapy in your own home would cost considerably less. No need for airfares or accommodation. Juicers and medication are available, and there is no need to lose dollars in the American exchange as we did. Let me give you a break down.

The full therapy at home initially cost approximately $300 per week. This cost included all the organic produce required (growing your own is much cheaper, an excellent reference source is "Organic Gardening" by Peter Bennet, ISBN 1-86436-043-7), all medication and supplements, water and sundries. Then there were several assisting therapies we took on which helped in the cleansing of the blood and built up my immune system. This added to our weekly cost accordingly. (approximately $150.00)

Don't be shy to ask for discounts when doing your buying. We did and the response was amazing.

Unlike the wealth of information we have gathered to pass onto you, we did not have the same pleasure, so I therefore packed my bags and delved into the unknown. I came back a winner!

Needless to say, this came about due to a great sacrifice. The business I had built up from nothing over the course of ten years had to be sold as I made perhaps the biggest decision of my life. As you can no doubt appreciate, this decision was not an easy one to make. Far from it. There were a lot of sorrowful feelings, but it was a matter of necessity, so therefore, emotion couldn't afford to play a part.

As time elapsed and the bills mounted, Anna and I decided to sell our house in order to keep up with our commitments and the costs of the ongoing therapy. A lot of emotion surfaced as we contemplated this sell-off of yet another one of our assets, but once again we could not allow emotions to cloud the issue. We had to get the mortgage out of the way!

Before the sell-off we drew on our superannuation fund which we had planned as our retirement nest egg.

To some, I guess, such developments would be met with horror. After all, in the society in which we live, material wealth appears to be the be-all and end-all of our existence. I had once adhered to this doctrine, but time and events have a way of changing one's perspective.

My present philosophy is: material wealth is obtainable if you want it. Health is an absolute necessity. Once it is lost, there is no guarantee of regaining it. This is a truth that should be self-evident, but somehow we have lost sight of this fundamental belief. It is essential to return to this maxim and not merely pay it lip service, but to actually LIVE IT!

I offer a word of advice to those who would treat their health as they would a material object. The time to look after your health is while you still have it.

THE GREAT IRONY

The great irony of course, is that if I had undertaken the orthodox treatment, it would have cost me $0. I'd probably have paid someone to look after my business for several months then returned back to work.

This option has cost me significantly financially. This is an immutable fact. The sacrifice in this area has been great. It has been a challenge to be sure, but one which I am prepared to meet head on. It is my conviction that it has all been worth it. Fortunately, I have had assets which allowed me to fund my therapy. Tragically, not everyone can do this, but then again, as Anna pointed out to me, although a great deal is spent on organic produce and medication, our outgoings for take-away, sweets, drinks and basically your everyday junk food have diminished, which she feels somehow balances up the score.

The bottom line is this — the toxic conventional treatments are free, the alternatives are not. Therefore there is not much of a choice for the majority of patients. The alternative treatment, so simplistic in its ideals and diet based, has to be funded out of the patient's own pocket.

There needs to be a revolutionary upheaval for this imbalance to be addressed. I feel with all my heart that this change is here.

It's already happening!

Just some of the subtle changes already apparent are the growing number of pharmacies stocking large varieties of vitamin and mineral supplements. Another is the number of people unhappy with their GPs, now seeking alternative therapies to cure their ailments via naturopaths and homeopaths.

The ever increasing number of organic shops appearing throughout the country, is an indication that people are becoming aware of the devastating effects of chemicals, artificial fertilizers and pesticides that are being used within our food industry.

As mentioned before, it is possible to undertake a partial detoxification programme as Anna did, by simply modifying your diet accordingly *(refer to Book Reviews, "GET A LIFE" by Kathryn Alexander, page 229)*.

ANOTHER MIRACLE

The following chapter details yet another miracle that can be attributed to the Gerson Therapy. It relates to the conception of our third child whom we affectionately refer to as our 'Organic Baby'.

Infertility

Anna and I had a plan for our lives together. We were to travel first, then settle down and have a family, beginning in 1988 when we returned from our overseas trip. This plan was scuttled when for a year, we had no result in becoming pregnant. A visit to Anna's gynaecologist resulted in us being referred to a specialist and then admitted to a fertility programme. This was brought about due to the fact that my previous tests had shown that I had a low sperm count and some sperm present were 'mutated', which means that some had no tail, whilst others had no head.

Call it the male ego, call it what you will, the bottom line was that this made me feel totally inadequate, 'subhuman' even. These feelings were compounded a great deal by what I perceived as a lack of compassion within the medical profession that we encountered. Needless to say, this greatly affected my psychological well-being. All they needed to say to me was, don't worry, there are thousands of cases like this and that you are not alone.

Added to all this was the fact that Anna had antibodies that wouldn't allow my sperm to do its job. She also had fluctuating hormonal levels occurring around her ovulation time. Taken cumulatively, these problems conspired to make natural conception impossible. By the time we underwent tests and actually started treatment, another year went by, bringing us to 1990.

Let me add at this point that the fertility programme is a very costly exercise because we saw many couples completely distraught after several failed attempts, they could simply not continue because of lack of money. We truly felt for these couples.

The AIH (Artificial Insemination by Husband) programme that Anna and I were undertaking was, as anyone who has experienced it can testify, a trying time. Every morning over a specified period of time, Anna would journey to the fertility clinic at 6.30 am to undergo hormone injections. Once her hormones were at a level conducive to conception, Anna would then be artificially inseminated.

Our first attempt at artificial insemination tragically ended in miscarriage. Picking ourselves up and dusting ourselves off, we persevered until finally, on 2/11/1991, we were gifted with a beautiful set of twins, Christian and Olivia. We now felt complete and relieved. After four years of pain and suffering, we produced two beautiful babies.

We were told that should we ever consider having more children, we would need to go back on the programme. Since we already had been blessed with two beautiful children, we did not consider this option. We did not want to go through the trying time again, so we decided our family was complete.

However in April 1996 Anna fell pregnant without medical intervention. Had I consented to radiotherapy, I would have been left sterile, therefore no more children. Another miracle! On New Year's Eve 1996, Anna gave birth to our little organic baby boy Lawrence (VICTORY!) — a bouncing 8 pounder!

This is undoubtedly the most beautiful chapter of the Gerson story, another victory to the man who dared to believe in his convictions and acted on them to produce pockets of happiness in this world.

Anna and I know it was the Gerson Therapy that helped us regain our fertility. *(See page 45 for the modified Gerson Therapy that Anna was using)*. We stand here, true testimony of the therapy, no matter what the ailment!

A network in development

Another true inspirational advocate of the Gerson way of life is Fabiola, a little girl who we befriended together with her mother Flora at the Gerson Clinic in Mexico in 1995.

FABIOLA

Her story is one of true courage and will to live. Fabiola was born in 10 April 1986. In July 1988 she was diagnosed with a malignant tumour on the right kidney. This subsequently led to her having four treatments of chemotherapy. In July 1988 the tumour along with the right kidney was removed, the tumour mass measured 17cm x 26cm. This again was followed by another four treatments of chemotherapy up to April 1989. Thereafter she maintained regular checks and analysis in the form of C.T. scans and blood tests. In 1991, when Fabiola underwent another C.T. scan, it was discovered that the cancer had spread to the liver and another operation followed. Her mother expressed to us her anger that in the two years when

Claudio, Fabiola, Martina and Flora

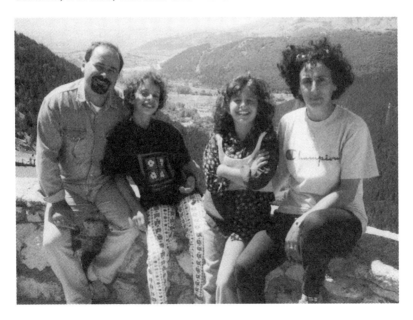

they were told she was all clear no advice was offered to them by the medical establishment regarding diet. They were told that she could eat whatever she liked.

Another operation was performed with the suggestion of another ten courses of chemotherapy to be undertaken over a 12 month period. As they had no other option, they decided to proceed. However, after her second course of chemotherapy, they decided to delve into alternative treatments. They went to a homeopath who adjusted Fabiola's diet and supplemented it with vitamins and minerals. A particular immune enhancer that Fabiola lives by and has helped her immensely throughout her battle is a substance called Germanium sesquioxide (*see Medication Table, page 241*). It helped her tremendously while she was undergoing chemotherapy. She never lost her appetite, in fact she actually put on weight. She did not require any blood transfusions, she never vomited and above all, she was always vivacious and happy and remains so.

In May 1992, further metastases were discovered, this time in the lungs. Her oncologist said she had three to four months survival, at best.

They returned to their homeopath, who prescribed various immune enhancing therapies for Fabiola. These combined therapies slowed the spread until September 1995, when further metastases were discovered in her diaphragm and one on her vertabrae.

On advice from their homeopath they went to Mexico and

underwent the Gerson Therapy where we met. We immediately formed a very strong bond as we were able to converse in the same language (Italian) and assisted them by interpreting their doctor's instructions.

Two years on and we still maintain regular contact with them, and are pleased to say that Fabiola is doing well and they are happy to say there seems to be no further spread. They live every day as it comes and are grateful for alternative therapies, for without them, Fabiola would not be here.

MEXICO

While in Mexico we befriended many people from many parts of the world, with many different problems, ranging from heroin addiction, diabetes, stroke, hepatitis to cancer and everything in between. One in particular, was a gentleman in his late sixties from Canada. He was diagnosed with Nephrotic Syndrome. He arrived at the Gerson Institute shortly before us and was confined to a wheelchair due to his deteriorated condition. Nephrotic Syndrome is a kidney disorder which results in an accumulation of fluid in the body tissues. His condition was so severe that he had been given only three weeks to live. He had gained in excess of 30kgs in fluid; he was literally drowning in his own body fluid. For two weeks we did not see him as he was confined to his room and we all feared the worst. However, on the third week, he emerged from his room, virtually unrecognisable. I mean this in a positive sense, for he had lost over 20kgs of body fluid and was full of life with no wheelchair in sight. Both he and his wife were overjoyed with the results and could not wait to return home to their family and see their doctor who had sent him home to die.

What truly inspired all of us at the Gerson Institute whilst we were there, was the presence of a young Academic Trauma Surgeon from Texas. His cancer was Ewing's Sarcoma. This is a highly malignant form of bone cancer mainly affecting children up to the age of 15, and very rare amongst adults. When I questioned him about orthodox medicine, he replied that it was not effective in the treatment of this particular cancer. I asked how he came across the Gerson Therapy. He said he found it on the Internet, and that it was the only scientifically validated therapy which showed some success in treating this type of cancer.

Unfortunately we have not been able to keep in touch with the above two, so we do not know their current progress.

ANNA

Another case that has been inspirational to us has been that of Anna. We first met her in early 1997. She had been diagnosed with an aggressive type of breast cancer which had spread to her bones and liver. Her prognosis was so bad that her doctor advised her to make out a will and to enjoy the remaining time she had left. She had heard of what I had been doing, and since she did not consider chemotherapy or radiation which had been suggested, an option, she came to see me.

She was prescribed hormone therapy to control and shrink the tumour in her breast, however this did not help in any way the cancer in her bones or liver.

I guided her through the Gerson therapy, including some other alternative therapies and she also sought alternative medical help and advice in the form of intravenous Vitamin C, Shark Cartilage, coffee enemas and mega doses of vitamin and mineral supplements. Her condition did not immediately improve and her blood was in such poor condition, that she needed a blood transfusion. Throughout her ordeal she suffered severe head and back aches.

Her condition was still very poor. It was then suggested she try the "Cancer Leukaemia, The Breuss Cancer Cure" (Australian School of Herbal Medicine, ISBN 0-646-34773-X) which involves cleansing the body of toxins via a radical fasting therapy. Throughout this therapy she vomited, had no energy to walk or shower on her own. During this period she would pray constantly.

After six weeks on the therapy, she began to regain her strength and appetite. It was at this point she required another blood transfusion. Nonetheless, she continued to improve dramatically. The lump under her arm had almost disappeared along with her head and back aches.

She has discontinued the hormone therapy and has no need for pain killers. She maintains a healthy organic diet and prays daily. Without the love and support from her daughters Theresa and Lina and other family members, Anna knows she would not have come this far.

BILL

Bill first had cancer in 1979 with Fourth Stage Non-Hodgkins Lymphoma. A big growth was at the back of his stomach and it was in the bones and blood as well. God's answer to his and wife Mary's question of "What do we do?" were the words "Pray, as much as possible". A friend was led to come and pray for Bill for one to two hours at a time on a regular basis. Also many other people were praying for Bill. This led to many beautiful spiritual experiences, and eventually to a very deep experience of inner healing, after which Bill rapidly started to put on weight and his cancer receded. As well as prayer, Bill had nine treatments of chemotherapy which doctors had said would not cure him, but might buy him some extra time.

The second time, 12 years later, Bill had a tumour in one lung and on one kidney, but the blood was not involved. Cancer was more virulent than the first time. This time they were led to go to the Hippocrates Health Centre in Queensland, to detoxify the body so it could cure itself. Also bill had a Stem Cell Transplant, which at the time was a new experimental process. He 'came good' again, to use an Australian expression.

The next time, in 1995, Bill developed a growth on the left side of his face. It looked like he had a toothache. At first, doctors thought looking at the scans, that cancer was all through his body, and were speaking to each other in hushed voices of palliative care. But what they saw on the scans turned out to be only the effects of the previous cancers, like scar tissue, so it was confined only to the face. This time a Naturopath told us about two cancer treatments, Shark Cartilage Powder and the Dr Hulda Clark Book "The Cure for All Cancer", a parasite eradication programme, both of which we followed. Bill also had Radiotherapy on the face, and used Shark Cartilage Cream to prevent the radiated area from staying brown, and it returned to normal.

As well as all this they read many books on cancer and health and healing, and all seemed to point to detoxifying the body and the soul, and to feed each with pure wholesome food, the soul with spiritual food, and the body with food as close to its natural state as possible. As God created it for us and as taught at the Hippocrates Health Centre.

Bill said in a recent talk, "three times I've had cancer, three times the doctors told me I was going to die, three times I didn't believe them, and to prove it, I'm still here".

ANGELA

Angela is 63 years old and her story starts in December 1996. After complaining of back pain, her daughter Maritsa took her to her local GP for a visit. Routine tests were set up for her in January 1997 which included blood and urine tests, X-rays, bone scans and a bone marrow biopsy.

In February 1997 they received her results when they visited the specialist. The result was Multiple Myeloma, a form of bone cancer.

At this stage the pain was very bad and she was prescribed a cocktail of drugs for her pain including oral morphine. The therapy first offered was a high dose of 'experimental double blood stem cell transplantation' followed by Interferon, Melphalan and Prednisolene (chemotherapy) every four weeks. This would have been followed by Adriamycin and Bleomycin for six weeks and oral Cyclophosphamide and Melphalan every six weeks. To say they were confused is an understatement.

Angela could not shower herself, she needed help dressing and even needed help getting in and out of bed. Even a task as simple as sitting had become painful. The painkillers she had started taking caused her constipation which added to her pain.

Angela with the support of her family, decided to take an alternative path. They consulted with doctors who dealt in this field. The first thing to do as with all other alternative therapies, was to change her diet and start supplement intake and enemas.

After a month, the pain eased considerably and in time the painkillers were no longer needed. As she started to improve, Angela started doing things for herself and she gained a new confidence and even stronger faith in God.

Unknowingly, in December 1997, she started having goats milk in her diet which unfortunately increased her protein levels and thus caused her pain to return. Since her protein levels were too high, her doctor put her on the Breuss Therapy for 42 days. She found it extremely hard the first three weeks but she soon started regaining her energy levels and her pain disappeared.

Her blood results in March 1998 following the diet, were very encouraging and her doctors were pleased with the results.

With a lot of love, patience, a supportive family, positive attitude, discipline and a deep faith in God, Angela took charge of her life and embarked on a plane in June 1998 for a visit to her birthplace in Cyprus.

DEAN

In February 1998, Dean went to see his local GP because he was overweight and feeling unwell. This visit resulted in a series of blood tests over the next two months. At first Glandular Fever was thought to have been the problem but subsequent blood tests suggested that he could possibly have Leukaemia.

After a bone marrow biopsy was arranged by his GP on 20 April, the results were confirmed by the specialist on 24 April that he did indeed have Chronic Lymphoid Leukaemia. A second opinion also confirmed the results.

The only good news given to him was that it was slow growing, but unfortunately no-one that had had it in the past lived for more than five years and they didn't know how long Dean had it for. The grim reality was that there was no 'medical cure' so in other words it was terminal.

Being from a Christian family, prayer played the most important part which gave him a positive attitude.

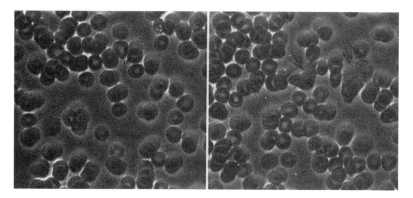

Before

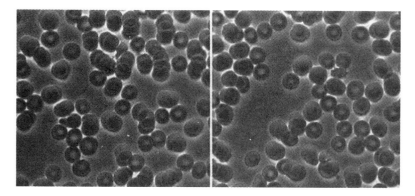

Taken approximately six weeks later

Dean first came upon the Breuss Therapy when visiting his local health store. He read the book by Rudolph Breuss and on 28 April he commenced the 42 day fast as well as visiting his naturopath who conducted a live blood analysis and provided him with vitamin and mineral supplements. He also had his home detoxified, as suggested in the book, from moth balls, nephthalene flakes, insects sprays etc.

Over the next two weeks, Dean continued to have special prayer meetings with his Pastor and friends, abiding strictly to his fast, despite his body aching and shaking constantly.

Although there were days he felt like giving up, the love and determination from his family members, got him through.

Dean currently feels and looks fantastic and although he believes he has been healed, he cannot claim a medical remission for five years. He continues to juice and eat fresh fruit, vegetables and nuts supplemented by vitamins and minerals every day. His blood results are excellent and with the help of God he claims not only remission but healing.

CORINNE

A copy of her letter:

I was originally diagnosed in October 1996 with a caecal carcinoma. As I had not been feeling well for some time and immediately before diagnosis had been in considerable pain I think I had some idea that something was very wrong and as such was not overly surprised at the diagnosis. During the previous couple of years I had also been under considerable stress at work and in my personal life and I feel that this contributed significantly to my health status. I underwent surgery to remove the growth and opted for a six month regime of chemotherapy as a safe-guard, as one Lymph node had shown some cancerous cells. As I'm usually a 'bite the bullet' and do what has to be done type of person I set my mind on what had to be done and did not really contemplate that this disease may develop into something much more serious or even life threatening.

At this stage the modifications I made to lifestyle centered around lessening some of my work pressure by becoming part time and reviewing work practices and expectations. I explored personal issues with a therapist and became kinder to myself accepting some faults etc. as OK. At this time I did not modify my diet very much although I did take naturopathic remedies and herbs to assist with side effects of chemotherapy and digestion problems. I finished chemotherapy and rejoiced in an all clear diagnosis.

Approximately two months later I started to experience pain soon after eating which continued to develop until exploratory surgery in December 1997 confirmed another mass higher in my abdomen on the superior mesenteric artery. Surgeons did not remove it as they felt it was too risky to remove, or if they were successful, would significantly compromise my quality of life. Radiotherapy was not an option due to risk to surrounding organs, and chemotherapy would involve a new drug with a very low success rate and dramatic side effects. WOW did this prognosis knock my socks off!! After a few weeks of tears, panic and feeling totally lost and helpless I remembered words attributed to Helen Keller "Life is a daring adventure or nothing". With this began the adventure of my lifetime.

This adventure has led me to meet many and varied people, read a myriad of books and explore every aspect of my life including diet and physical health, spirituality, relationships and my emotional well being. I opted not to have chemotherapy and to look at natural ways to assist my body to heal. I took extended leave from work to enable me to concentrate on all aspects of healing my body and soul. I started by using relaxation techniques and meditation to calm my inner self which have been fantastic. I have not been a particularly religious person but view myself as a spiritual person.

I started to read, discuss and deepen this aspect of my life looking to my connectedness to all mankind, the power in the universe, that in fact we are a soul with a body rather than a body with a soul and how to nurture that soul. Deepening this aspect of my life has added a new dimension to life and brought an inner peace and calmness. I have pursued personal work in the areas of forgiveness, giving and receiving unconditional love and looking at how attitudes and thoughts dramatically effect the way I function and my perspective on life and illness. This has certainly helped me gain perspective on what is important in life and rejuvenated my sense of fun and mischief. I now live, enjoy and rejoice in the beauty of each day. I find that living by the principle that life should be treasured and enjoyed, that each obstacle is an opportunity to learn something new, and that every moment should be enjoyed for what it is, not wasted away on worries, or in the rush toward, or fear of what the future holds. A smile and a laugh is priceless.

Modification of diet has also been an important part of my healing process. Much reading and discussion with many people has led me to a natural fresh diet with few refined foods, chemicals, preservatives etc. Many 'cancer' beating diets have been written about but I think the most important factor is to find one, or combine factors of all, to develop one that suits you and then to enjoy what you do eat! A friend recently mentioned the Breuss 42 day Juice fast. As a large proportion of my diet had already comprised of fresh juices, and fasts have been used in Europe for many years for various health reasons, I thought I'd give it a go. It also sounded like a great way to detoxify the body.

Well what an interesting exercise that proved to be! There were several ups and downs during the fast. Unlike others on the fast I was ravenously hungry for five weeks with the hunger only disappearing in the last week. Surprisingly my weight dropped very little although I certainly had weight I could lose. Initially my energy levels surged, then dropped dramatically, then resumed to a heightened level in the week after completion. There were a couple of teary days where my emotions seemed to be all over the place and exploration of this with a counsellor helped identify issues and beliefs in relation to food which were being challenged by being on the fast. This was of immense benefit to me in relation to my further modification of diet and understanding what and why I eat and how this subsequently affects my health and healing. I was progressing reasonably well until the three week mark when I ran into some physiological problems with my stomach and bowel. I was not being supervised during the fast and so modified the fast to include a few mouthfuls of boiled potato skin each day which alleviated the problem. Discussion with a naturopath since has identified a different course of action I could have taken without eating. If undertaking a fast again I would not do so without over-seeing of a medical or natural therapist. I opted to continue the modified fast to completion of the 42 days. Although not mentioned in the fast regime I also undertook a daily coffee enema. This appeared to help immensely in the detoxification process as I always felt considerably 'cleaner and less toxic' with increased energy afterwards.

I did not find this an easy regime to do, nor was it intolerable. Boy do you notice how many food advertisements are on TV!!! The people doing it at the same time as me all differed in how difficult or easy they found the fast, obviously a unique experience for each individual. I had great love and support from family and friends which certainly helped me get through the tough times. I would suggest that anyone attempting the fast should ask their family to cook their own meals!. Although I ran into some physiological difficulties and needed to modify the fast I feel it was of great benefit to me. My live blood culture showed an improvement from start to finish and some evidence of healing was present. Scans before and after showed that although the cancer does not appear to have shrunk it also hadn't grown — A great start in the healing process! Through the fast people commented on how well I looked, my skin and eyes were much clearer, my pain level decreased dramatically and I generally felt very well. In fact in the last few weeks I felt better than I had for a considerable period of time. I will probably undertake a shorter fast in the future as I feel this a beneficial process. With love, laughter, and light I wish you well in your life's adventure — May you feel peace and happiness.

Corinne

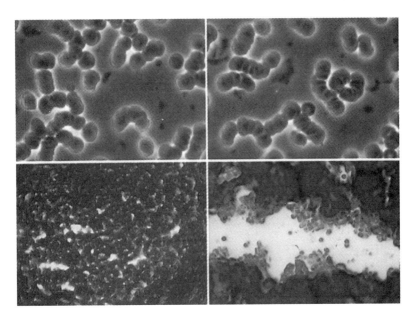

Blood taken 1/5/98

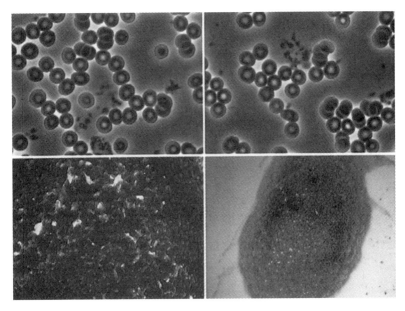

Blood taken 12/6/98

THE THERAPY

In this chapter I will outline the therapy step by step, the way we undertook it in Mexico. Several topics are covered again, such as enemas, juicers and recipes. I stress to anyone wishing to undertake the therapy, to purchase a copy of "A CANCER THERAPY", by Max Gerson, MD and consult with a GP who is conversant with the Gerson Therapy. *(The publication is available from Inner Glow, page 88.)*

Routine

6.00 am   Coffee enema

7.00 am   Liver and B12 injection

8.00 am   *Breakfast*
                 1 glass orange juice: with 1 teaspoon potassium compound solution *(refer to page 241)* and 3 drops of Lugol's solution in juice, together with 2 acidol pepsin, 1 thyroid, 1 niacin and pancreatin. *(see medication table, page 241)*.
                 Oatmeal porridge: with stewed fruits and honey and piece of fruit.

9.00 am   Carrot juice (1 glass: 6 medium sized carrots)

9.30 am   Green juice (1 glass: 1 small apple, piece of green capsicum, several leaves of endive, watercress, cos lettuce, beetroot leaves) a combination of all. 1 teaspoon potassium compound solution in juice.

10.00 am   Carrot and apple juice (1 glass: 3 medium sized carrots to one medium sized apple) together with 1 thyroid, 1 niacin and 2 CoQ10. 1 teaspoon potassium compound solution and 3 drops Lugol's solution in juice.
            Coffee enema
            Plate of fresh fruit

11.00 am   Carrot juice (1 glass) with 2 liver capsules

12.00 pm   Green juice (1 glass) 1 teaspoon potassium compound solution.

1.00 pm   *Lunch*
            Carrot juice (1 glass) with 2 acidol pepsin, 1 thyroid, 1 niacin, 3 pancreatin, 2 CoQ10.
            Hippocrates soup, baked potato with crushed garlic and one tablespoon flax seed oil, green salad with diluted red wine vinegar and baked or boiled vegetables. Fresh fruit.

2.00 pm   Green juice (1 glass). 1 teaspoon potassium compound solution in juice.

3.00 pm   Carrot juice (1 glass with 2 liver capsules).
            Fresh fruit platter

4.00 pm   Carrot and apple juice (1 glass with 2 liver capsules). 1 teaspoon potassium compound solution and 3 drops Lugol's solution in juice.

5.00 pm   Carrot and apple juice (1 glass with 1 thyroid, 1 niacin, 3 pancreatin). 1 teaspoon potassium compound solution and 3 drops Lugol's solution in juice.

6.00 pm   Green juice (1 glass with 1 niacin, 2 CoQ10). 1 teaspoon potassium compound solution in juice.

7.00 pm   *Dinner*
           Carrot juice (1 glass with 2 acidol pepsin, 1 thyroid, 1 niacin, 3 pancreatin).
           Hippocrates soup, baked potato with crushed garlic and 1 tablespoon flax seed oil, salad, vegetables and fresh fruit.

10.00 pm   Coffee enema.

GIVING INJECTIONS

With the Gerson diet, B12 is lacking, and therefore needs to be taken in supplemental form.

B12 is readily available by prescription from your local GP. We were shown how to prepare and self-administer these injections by a registered nurse.

HOURLY SCHEDULE FOR PATIENT ON THE GERSON THERAPY ①

John Gerson

Change after 3-4 weeks. ② ⑯
For non malignant diseases see Appendix (1)

Start Date:
Change Date:

Name:

TIME	③ ⑪ JUICES 8 OZ. EACH	③ DIET	Flax seed oil Tbsp p.246	④ Acidoll Pepsin, caps.	MEDICATION							⑪ Injection, 100 mcg B-12 combined with 3cc liver	⑫ Coffee Enemas	⑫ Castor Oil Treatment	⑬ Tests
					⑤ Potassium Compound Solution, teaspoons in juice	⑥ Lugol 1/2 Strength, drops in juice	⑦ Thyroid 1 gr. tabl.	⑧ Niacin 50 mg. tabl.	⑨ Pancreatin tabl.	⑩ LIVER Caps.					
8:00	Orange	Breakfast		2	1	3	1	1	3		ONCE DAILY	Every 4 hours or more as needed	Every other day	Complete blood count; Serum electrolytes; Urinalysis.
9:00	Green				1									
9:30	Apple-carrot				1	3								
10:00	Apple-carrot				1	3	1	1						
11:00	Carrot			NO MEDICATION										
12:00	Green				1									
1:00	Apple-carrot	Lunch		2	1	3	1	1	3	2				
2:00	Green				1									
3:00	Carrot			NO MEDICATION										
4:00	Carrot			NO MEDICATION							2			
5:00	Apple-carrot				1	3	1	1	3	2				
6:00	Green				1									
7:00	Apple-carrot	Dinner		2	1	3	1	1	3					

INNER GLOW / GERSON SUPPORT NETWORK

Inner Glow Products: PO Box 162 Tewantin QLD 4565 (Noosa Shire), Australia. Fax: (07) 5449 0900 or 5449 0600. Inner Glow offers support to Gerson patients along with books, audio tapes, videos, juicers, enema kits, etc. We have personally found them to be very helpful and knowledgeable in the Gerson Therapy.

Acidol pepsin: Aids digestion. Taken prior to meals.
Thyroid: Helps correct an imbalanced metabolism. (Discontinue during menses).
Niacin: Necessary for the body's energy metabolism and for the synthesis of fatty acids. (May cause hot, red skin. This is temporary and harmless. Discontinue during menses or in a case of haemorrhage).
Lugol's solution: To restore the loss of iodine.
Potassium Compound Powder: To restore the imbalance between sodium and potassium levels within the cells. Brought over from the United States in 100g bottles. This needs to be diluted into 900ml of distilled water and kept in the fridge *(For further information, refer to page 241)*.

FOOD

The following was our weekly grocery list whilst on the full Gerson Therapy:

To make the required juices, salads and soups, we use 23kg of carrots, 18kg of apples, (preference granny smith apples when available) 7 green capsicums and approximately 14 lettuce, 20kg of potatoes,11kg of onions, and 9kg of tomatoes. Other fruits and vegetables are bought as we require them.

The first six to eight weeks of the therapy are very strict and basically a vegan diet. After this period I introduced different foods such as yoghurt, fish, brown rice, pasta, legumes and breads. All of these in moderation and organic where possible. When buying fish, we only buy deep sea fish because they contain minimal pollutants and are highly mineralized.

I eat a variety of vegetables and fruits except for mushrooms, pineapples, cucumbers, avocados and all berries, which are not allowed on the diet. Salt is definitely forbidden as is nicotine, sweets, coffee, sugar, alcohol, bottled, canned, preserved or frozen food. (Refer to "A CANCER THERAPY", by Max Gerson.)

When cooking meals, we only use either stainless steel or cast iron pots. The latter I highly recommend, as they require very little water when cooking and retain all the natural flavours and nutrients of the vegetables. Teflon is also allowed as long as it isn't damaged. Absolutely no aluminium is allowed. The most important thing is that the pots have tight fitting lids allowing minimal evaporation.

We also went through a large quantity of coffee, not for drinking of course, for enemas. It is important that the coffee is organic. It can be bought in beans or already ground. It is available at organic stores, some health stores and some coffee houses.

A particular brand we have been extremely pleased with and recommend is "Paradiso" organically grown coffee, medium roast, filter fine, ground and available in 250 gm packs. It is available from most organic stores, or you can write to: Arabicas Pty Ltd, PO Box 680, Goroka, Papua New Guinea. Tel: 7321272 or 7322496, Fax: 7322949.

Two teas which we enjoy are camomile and peppermint. Camomile is calming, alkalising, settles the tummy and is great for the kidneys. I am always assured a restful night's sleep with camomile tea. Peppermint, in particular, I enjoy the most as it is not only refreshing to the palate but also assists in digestion. Excellent for nausea. There are many other herbal teas available, it's just a matter of taste.

Recipes for the patient undergoing the Gerson Therapy

OATMEAL

Pour 1 cup of rolled oats into a stainless steel pot, add enough water to cover the oats and let sit overnight. The following morning just heat and stir to desired consistency.

STEWED FRUIT

We add a combination of dried fruits to our porridge and prepare them as above eg. Add a handful of raisins and apricots, several prunes and peaches into a stainless steel pot and cover with water. As with the oats, we let the fruit sit overnight so they absorb as much water as possible. We heat them at the same time as the oats and let boil for several minutes. Drain off excess water and add to oats. (Enough for 2 people).

HIPPOCRATES SOUP

Boil one litre of water and add two scrubbed and quartered potatoes, 2 diced sticks of celery, 1 diced leek, 2 cut tomatoes and a little parsley. Cook slowly for approximately 2 hours, then put through food mill. Alternatively, you can dice all your vegetables and eat them as a minestrone. *We prefer to use either distilled (food grade) or spring water for cooking and drinking.*

BAKED POTATO

Insert a metal skewer through the potato (or slit) and bake for about 1 hour. Never use alfoil to wrap the potato when cooking.

CALF'S LIVER

Calf's liver is an important part of the Gerson Therapy. However, because of diminishing supplies of organic calf's liver, desiccated liver supplements together with B12 and Crude Liver Extract, and high dosages of carrot juice, were used instead.

We have found that the best source to attain calf's liver is from dairy farms. These we located through BFA and NASAA. Their phone numbers are:

BFA: Biological Farmers Association. Tel: 076 393 299

NASAA: National Association for Sustainable Agriculture Australia. Tel: 8370 8455

For preparation of the liver juice, refer to "A CANCER THERAPY" by Max Gerson.

FLAX SEED OIL

Available from organic and health stores, this oil is the richest source of valuable omega-3, -6 & -9 fatty acids. Flax oil contains almost twice as much nutrients than fish oils, which clinically have proven to benefit a number of health conditions, cancer being one of them. The oil has a nutty taste to it and tastes great on baked potatoes and salads. This oil should never be fried or cooked with and always store in the refrigerator for a maximum of 4-6 weeks after opening.

WATER

Water is a big issue. It is imperative to have only the purest water available. Through experience we have gained valuable knowledge regarding water purification. Distillation produces by far the purest water. Reverse osmosis is also a very effective means of water purification. For more information refer to the "The Water You Drink" by Jonathan Archer (*Book Reviews, page 216*) Home distilled water (not car battery distilled water) is essential for re-hydration and detoxification. The "more empty" the water is, the stronger its capacity to draw toxins from the cells for elimination to the outside. Distillation is a method of purification where water is heated until it vapourises. As the water turns to steam, bacteria, minerals, and most other substances are left behind. The steam then cools and recondenses into relatively pure water. There are a variety of water distillers available varying in holding capacity, from 10.5L-200L.

Reverse Osmosis is another purification method used extensively. This method is effective in removing most contaminants and undesirable elements from water, however it is not as effective as distillation.

NB. Be wary of advertised under the sink water purification units, which sell for between $100 and $400. A reputable reverse osmosis unit will cost approximately $800.

ENEMAS

The therapy consists of two basic essential components. They are nourishment and detoxification. One without the other does not work effectively to achieve complete regeneration of cells. Some of the questions asked regarding the enemas are:

Q: *"What is an enema?"*
A: Full scientific explanation The Coffee Enema *(page 98)*.

Q: *"Is it really necessary?"*
A: Yes. It is essential in removing toxins from the body.

Q: *"How can I benefit from having an enema?"*
A: The most immediate benefit will be the sensation of feeling light and refreshed. The positive benefit knowing that the toxins are being released.

Q: *"Is it painful?"*
A: No. It is totally painless if done correctly, and in actual

fact is used for the relief of pain. It is also beneficial for constipation and the relief of migraines. Unlike commercial laxatives and medications, there are no side effects and no dependency. Through past experience even haemorrhoids disappear after several enemas.

Q: *"Are they harmful?"*
A: If prepared and administered correctly they are totally harmless. In the first three months of therapy, I self-administered 455 enemas with only positive effects.

Q: *"Are they easy to prepare?"*
A: Yes. For full details on preparation, *refer to page 88.* Enema Kits are available from Inner Glow, *page 88.*

CLAY PACKS

Clay packs or poultices, are made up of a soft composition of clay, usually heated and spread on a cloth and applied to the sore area of the body. The clay used is not the same as that used for sculpting. It is called by various names, the one we used in Mexico is called ionic clay. The clay has an adsorbing (not absorbing) effect like that of charcoal and aids detoxification. It is very helpful for ailments such as diarrhoea, poison, gastrointestinal problems and inflammation. Whilst in Mexico, a clay poultice was applied daily to my tumour.

The following are required to make up the poultice:

1. *Enough hot water to mix needed amount of clay powder as a paste.*
2. *Apply quickly to a square of clean muslin to prevent cooling.*
3. *Place over the area to be treated.*
4. *Cover with some plastic and wool cloth.*
5. *Bandage or pin in place and leave on overnight.*

Recently I have become aware of an ionic clay, similar in its drawing powers to the one we used at the clinic, being used in body wraps. 'The Universal Contour Wrap', is a procedure whereby bandages are soaked in warm sea clay then applied to the body by wrapping them around the entire body, starting from the ankles to the neck and even under the chin. A full body wrap is an effective way to firm, tone and cleanse the body and skin from the toxins as well as losing centimetres. Anna actually went along and had three sessions, to verify its potential drawing benefits, as well as enjoying centimetre loss, and found it truly to be beneficial. She immediately found relief in her neck and shoulders on her first visit, where she always tends to accumulate toxins. Overall she found it very relaxing and enjoyable. The whole procedure takes approximately two hours from start to finish.

For further information about the wraps or ionic clay you can contact 'Totally U' at PO Box 360, Black Rock Victoria 3193, Australia. Tel: (03) 9521 8055.

CASTOR OIL PACKS

I found castor oil packs, to be most beneficial when I experienced pain, such as abdominal pain. It is also very soothing for people suffering with painful joints, in particular arthritis.

Procedure:

1. *Soak 3 pieces of white flannel with castor oil and squeeze out excess.*
2. *Place flannel over affected area.*
3. *Place slightly larger sheet of plastic over the flannel.*
4. *Use Medium temperature heating pad or hot water bottle over area. Don't let the pack get cold or uncomfortably hot.*
5. *Keep on 1-1.5 hours; apply every four hours. You can re-use the castor oil pack.*

GRUEL

We had never heard of gruel before, but is has been around for a very long time. It is merely a by-product of oatmeal and is used to assist in nausea and vomiting. Its effect is instantaneous if the nausea is fairly mild but continuous consumption of the gruel throughout the nausea, will help settle the symptoms. It is also very nutritious and simple to make. It can be kept hot in a thermos for up to 10 hours. I would regularly sip a cup of gruel when feeling ill.

To make, simply add 1 cup of rolled oats into a saucepan and cover with 4 cups of water, bring to boil and stir gently for several minutes. Pour off liquid into a cup, leaving the rolled oats in the saucepan. The liquid has the consistency of coconut milk. In the early stages of the therapy, Anna would cook the oatmeal for breakfast and strain the gruel into a thermos.

I had been offered gruel at the clinic in Mexico but would never venture to try it, until one day when Anna was advised to take some herself. To her surprise the gruel was quite tasty, hence I started drinking it myself. If it wasn't for Anna, I would not have tried many of the foods or teas. She truly inspired me to try everything and urged me to enjoy it.

THE COFFEE ENEMA

The first time I ever came across an enema was when I was in Mexico. Believe me, I was not given instructions or told the procedure. Soon after our arrival, a nurse came into our room and told me to lie down on the bench which Anna had so meticulously laid out our suitcases and sorted out our belongings for the next four weeks. What she had thought was a towel rail was to be where I would be hanging up my enema bucket. She had truly thought the bench was for suitcases as you would expect to find in a hotel. Anyway after laying down on my right side, the nurse told me to pull down my pants and away we went for my first enema. Let me tell you, that first experience truly came as a shock, especially because the nurse tried to explain to us in broken English what she was doing and that future enemas would be administered by myself. After the initial shock, the enemas were a breeze and the benefits fully realised within a few days.

Unlike myself or many others who learnt about the coffee enema that way, I am going to outline exactly how the coffee enema is made, how often, the benefits, the history of the coffee enema and some extracts from newsletters we received from the Gerson Institute.

The first contact Dr Gerson had with coffee enemas was a medical paper he had read about their use in World War One. The facts are that wounded soldiers were in severe pain and due to the fact that the only morphine available was spared for surgery, the only other supply in abundance was coffee, which was used to keep the doctors awake for hours on end to tend the incoming wounded. A nurse for no apparent reason poured some coffee that was left in a pot into an enema bucket and instilled it into several patients for she could no longer bear their cries of pain. She noted that after several of these enemas the soldiers pain started to subside and indeed they started to improve. She reported this improvement to the head surgeon who immediately started the enemas with all other soldiers.

To think that something as simple as coffee can bring such relief in such severe cases within a short time! The following is an extract in part from a Gerson Institute Newsletter written by Gar Hildenbrand, June 1986.

A coffee enema!

NOW I'VE HEARD EVERYTHING.
WHAT DOES IT DO? HOW DOES IT WORK?

It is difficult to describe the incredulous facial expressions which ripple across a medical school lecture audience as the topic of coffee enemas is introduced. Embarrassed sniggering is heard from several seats in the hall.

A wise guy heckles, "How do you take it?" Charlotte Gerson

replies "Black — without cream and sugar." Laughter relaxes the entire room and Gerson goes on to explain this aspect of her famous father's (Max Gerson, MD) treatment: 3 tablespoons of regular grind organic coffee, boiled in a quart of distilled water for 3 minutes, covered and simmered for ten minutes, cooled to body temperature, filtered, and admitted to the colon using a short tip while lying on the right side. This is held for 12-15 minutes and released.

Responses from the audience are typical: "Boy, I'll bet you get a buzz out of that!" "Couldn't you just drink three or four cups of coffee?" And the eventual 'big question' is "What does it do?" "Why go to all that trouble just for a caffeine high?"

The coffee enema is, without question, the most unusual part of Gerson's combined regime and often evokes astonishment and mirth in persons who have never experienced an enema and who emphatically prefer to drink their coffee. Practitioners and patients who have had experience with coffee enemas, however, know that they are far more than a means of introducing stimulating caffeine into the bloodstream. From the patient's point of view, the coffee enema means relief from depression, confusion, general nervous tension, many allergy related symptoms and, most importantly, relief from severe pain.

In 1981, writing in Medical Hypotheses, Mark F. McCarty pointed out that "At a Senate Select Subcommittee hearing on cancer research in 1946, five independent MDs who had had personal experience with patients treated by Gerson, submitted letters indicating that they had been surprised and encouraged by the results they had seen, and urged a widespread trial of the method. One of these doctors claimed that relief of severe pain was achieved in about 90% of cases. No controlled trial of Gerson's methods has ever been undertaken."

The coffee enema has a very specific purpose: lowering serum toxins. (These are toxins within the blood) Dr Peter Lechner, who is currently conducting a trial of the Gerson cancer therapy in the post surgical treatment of liver metastasised colorectal cancers under the aegis of the Landeskrankenhaus of Graz, Austria, reported in 1984, "Coffee enemas have a definite effect on the colon which can be observed with an endoscope. Wattenberg and co-workers were able to prove in 1981 that the palmitic acid found in coffee promotes the activity of glutathione S-transferase and other ligands by manifold times above the norm. It is this enzyme group which is responsible primarily for the conjugation of free electrophile radicals which the gall bladder will then release.

Editors of Physiological Chemistry and Physics stated "Caffeine enemas cause dilation of bile ducts, which facilitates excretion of toxic cancer breakdown products by the liver and dialysis of toxic products from blood across the colonic wall."

In the late 1970s and early 1980s, researchers in the lab of Lee Wattenberg identified salts of palmitic acids (kahweol and cafestol palmitate) in coffee as potent enhancers of glutathione S-transferase, a major detoxification system that catalyses the binding of a vast variety of electrophiles from the blood stream to the sulfhydryl group of glutathione. Because the reactive ultimate carcinogenic forms of chemicals are electrophiles, the glutathione S-transferase system must be regarded as an important mechanism for carcinogen detoxification.

With this rationale in mind, we can expand on Gerson's hypothesised physiological actions and effects of coffee enemas. Gerson wrote that Heubner and Meyer of Geottingen University, Germany, had shown in animal models that rectal administration of caffeine would dilate bile ducts and promote bile flow. The introduction of a quart of coffee solution into the colon will dilute portal blood and, subsequently, the bile. Theophylline and theobromine, major constituents of coffee, dilate blood vessels and counter inflammation of the gut. The palmitates of coffee enhance glutathione S-transferase which is responsible for the removal of many toxic radicals from serum. Finally, the fluid of the enema itself stimulates the visceral nervous system promoting peristalsis and the transit of diluted toxic bile from the duodenum and out the rectum. Because the stimulating enema is retained for 15 minutes, and because all the blood in the body passes through the liver nearly every three minutes, these enemas represent a form of dialysis of blood across the gut wall.

It is obvious in light of the above that oral administration of beverage coffee cannot have the same effect. On the contrary, it virtually ensures re absorption of toxic bile.

As a medication, the coffee enema is in a class by itself. While other agents classed as choleretics do increase bile flow from the liver, they do little to enhance detoxifying enzyme systems, and they do not ensure the passage of bile from the intestines out the rectum. Bile is normally re-absorbed up to 9 or 10 times before working its way out the intestines in faeces. The enzyme enhancing ability of the coffee enema is unique among choleretics. Because it does not allow re-absorption of toxic bile by the liver across the gut wall, it is an entirely effective means of detoxifying the blood stream through existing enzyme systems in the liver and small bowel. Because clinical practice has shown coffee enemas to be well tolerated by patients when used as frequently as every four hours, the coffee enema may be classed as the only non-reabsorbed, effective, repeatable choleretic in the medical literature.

These enemas are safe when used within the context of the combined regime of Gerson. It is apparent that Gerson's intention in supplying a sodium restricted, high potassium, high micro-nutrient diet of fruits, vegetables and whole grains, was to supply all nutrients, known and unknown, which are necessary for cell respiration and energy production. High potassium, low sodium environments tend to return cell macromolecules to normal configuration states and to improve water structuring and water content. The addition by Gerson of supplemental salts of potassium (acetate, gluconate, and phosphate monobasic) to the diet in which malate is supplied by frequent use of apples probably greatly improves the efficiency of the Kreb's cycle in mitochondrial energy production. Protein restriction, employed by Gerson as a temporary aspect of treatment, has been observed empirically since before the turn of the century to aid in the reduction of cellular oedema. Administration of high Lugol's solution (iodine and potassium iodide in dilute solution) probably result in multiplication of mitochondria, which have their own DNA and RNA and replicate independently of the cell. Additionally, thyroid is known to enhance cell oxidation of sugars and therefore ATP production. In this way cell energy production is probably markedly increased.

Through these mechanisms, the therapy of Dr Max Gerson appears to:

a) reduce serum toxins to eliminate chronic challenge to damaged normal cells,
b) improve cell potassium ion content,
c) reduce cell sodium content,
d) reduce cell swelling through improved water structuring,
e) increase cell mitochondria count and activity, and
f) supply micro nutrients necessary for cell energy production and repair.

The contribution of low serum toxin levels by regular administration of coffee enemas is basic to increased cell energy production, enhanced tissue integrity, improved circulation, improved immunity, and improved tissue repair and regeneration which have been observed clinically to result from the administration of the combined regime of Gerson.

The bottom line is that enemas work effectively against reducing pain and eliminating toxic substances in our bodies.

Preparing a coffee enema

1 Enema bucket or douche set with nelaton catheter (available from Inner Glow, refer to page 88).

Ground certified organic coffee (available in beans or ground from health stores).

Distilled or spring water.

Vaseline, KY jelly or paw paw cream.

PROCEDURE (This is how <u>we</u> prepare our enema)

We boil one litre of water in a stainless steel pot. Then add three rounded tablespoons of ground organic coffee, stir and cover. Simmer for 10 minutes. We then filter the coffee into an enema bucket, making sure it is at body temperature (38°C). Several good filters we use are unbleached coffee bags, muslin cloths or a stainless steel tea strainer. We add pre-boiled distilled or spring water to the coffee to make up the loss of water through evaporation.

Once the enema is at the appropriate temperature, the valve clip is opened to let the coffee flow down the tube into a basin or trough. This is done so as no air will enter the colon.

Lying on our right side on a bench or floor, we draw our knees towards our chest, lubricating the tip of the nelaton catheter and inserting it approximately 6cm into the rectum. The enema bucket needs to be approximately 20cm above head height for the flow of coffee to be adequate. Once instilled, we shut off the valve clip and remove the catheter. We remain lying on our right side for approximately 12-15 minutes before releasing the enema. The first few times we found it difficult to retain the enema for the time required however, our endurance improved with time. The use of a kitchen timer is handy because it eliminates the need for clock-watching. This is a perfect time to practice meditation skills.

Once the enema is totally released, we ensure that our buckets are thoroughly cleaned with hot clean water, mild soap and hydrogen peroxide which we purchase from any supermarket or pharmacy (3%, 6% or 20% solution).

Some helpful hints to pass on from my experience follows:

1. When making the enema, instead of making one at a time, we make enough (as a concentrate) to last for the day. We can store it in the fridge, warming it as we need it.

2. We apply either vaseline, KY jelly or papaw cream to the tip of the catheter so it can easily slide into the rectum.

3. When cleaning our buckets, we use only distilled or spring water, the hotter the better. The soap we use is Camomile Kitchen Liquid Organic Cleaner which we dilute. This product and other organic products are available from Tri Nature and available only from distributors. Their

Various enema kits

*Enema Kits are available from Inner Glow Products
(see page 88)*

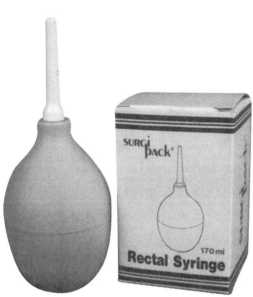

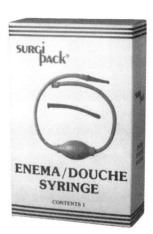

Enema Bag

For the administration of enemas or medications.

1.5 litre capacity with press lock closure, 1.5 m tube with open catheter tip

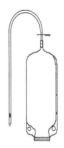

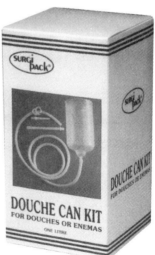

address is Box 304, Hunter Region Mail Centre NSW 2310. Tel: (049) 282 199, Fax: (049) 282 405 and they will inform you of your nearest distributor.

4. In the final rinse, we add one capful of Hydrogen Peroxide 3% or 6% food grade solution, which is available from pharmacies and supermarkets.

Believe me when I say it's not hard, it's just a matter of getting used to. Once you get past your first few, it'll be a breeze.

Castor Oil Enema

When preparing our castor oil enemas, we warm 2 tablespoons of castor oil in a glass standing in a pot of boiling water. We then pour the oil into the enema bag ensuring the oil slides down the tube. Once there is enough oil in the tube we shut off the valve and proceed to add either coffee or water as per our usual enema.

Have a good coffee break!

JUICERS

Juices are an essential part of the therapy and require a good juicer able to produce a high concentration of living enzymes, vitamins and minerals. Centrifugal juicers tend to oxidise and spoil the juice in a short time. There are machines designed to overcome this problem.

Over the past four years we have researched and experimented with different types of juicers and juice extractors. To date we have made over 5,500 juices, and spent over $5,000 on these different machines. I suppose this makes us somewhat juicing junkies. The following is a brief summary of three popular non centrifugal juicers we used.

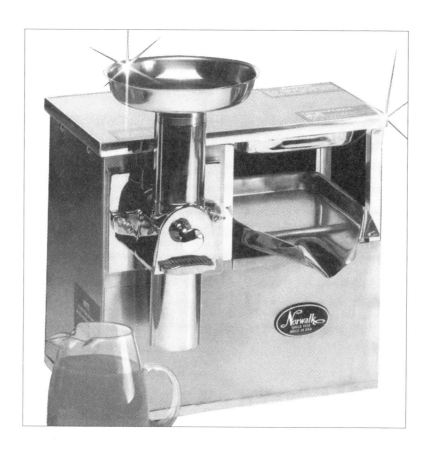

Norwalk Juicer

(We paid just under $4000 including import duties, and transportation from the USA in 1995).

The Norwalk was used at the Gerson Institute to make our juices. This juicer is by far the best as it grinds and presses separately, thereby extracting a higher concentration of living enzymes, vitamins and minerals from the juice.

For more information, contact
Norwalk Juicers
145 E.Cliff Street, Solana Beach CA 92075, USA
Tel: 0011-1-619 755 8423

Comments: We used the Norwalk juicer for the first six months of the therapy, and made just over 2,300 juices with it. The quality of juice is simply second to none and our family is living proof as to its positive effects.

The Norwalk is quite unique to any other juicer in that it grinds the produce to a pulp into a special filter bag. This bag is then folded and placed under the hydrolic press. The final product is a juice full of living enzymes, minerals and vitamins rich in flavour.

Cleaning the juicer is simple, a little extra time is needed to scrub and boil the filter bags, which then need to be placed in the freezer in readiness for the next juice.

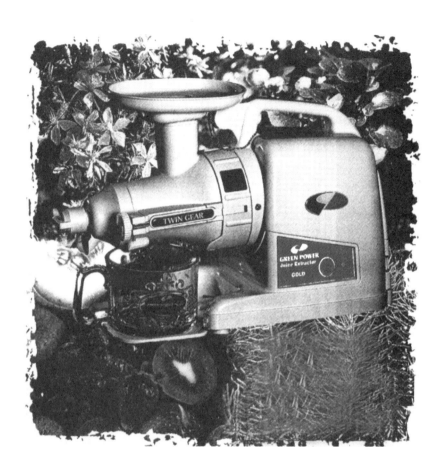

Green Power Juicer

(We paid $920, plus postage)

The Green Power Juicer is similar in size and shape to the Champion. It incorporates both infra red and ionisation technologies which allows the juice to retain its delicate balance of nutrients and enzymes whilst depositing heavy metals and pesticides in the pulp.

The Green Power Juicer is available from:

Living Proof
PO Box 377, Magill SA 5072, Australia
Tel: (08) 8364 4925

Comments: We found this particular machine produces a juice very similar in taste to the Norwalk. This leads me to believe it may contain similar portions of enzymes, vitamins and minerals. There is one considerable difference in that it doesn't require a press, therefore saving time, and no need to clean filter bags. This machine is by far the most efficient at producing 'green juices' eg. wheat grass, lettuce, spinach etc.

Much like the Norwalk, the Green Power is an extremely well made machine. However, we found this machine did require extra cleaning time compared to the others.

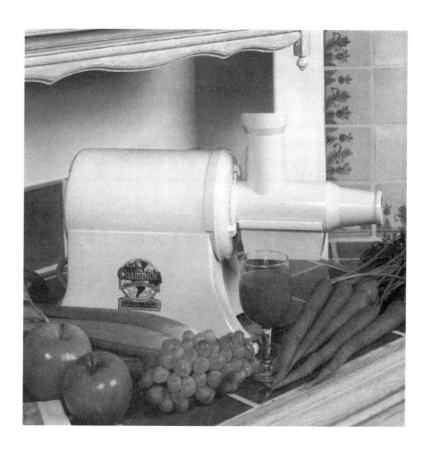

Champion Juicer

(We paid just under $500, including delivery)

This juicer is by far the most popular. Not only because of it's affordable price tag, but because it is simple to use and clean, while still retaining a high concentration of live enzymes, vitamins and minerals.

All enquiries and orders:

Living Proof

PO Box 377, Magill South Australia 5072

Tel: (08) 8364 4925

The Champion also comes with a sieve for those requiring a pulp free juice.

We were once told by an authority on the subject that the best juice comes by taking the pulp produced by the Champion and pressing it in a press similar to that of the Norwalk.

A word of advice to those who have limited hand movement, ie. arthritis. You may wish to start off with the Champion, as this would have to be the easiest to clean and operate.

Norwalk Juicer Order Form :

Dr. Norman Walker's Famous Hydraulic-Press Juicer is available to you **Factory Direct** . When you purchase a **Norwalk Juicer** you are investing in your health and the health of your family, a wise choice compared to the cost of items like furniture, televisions, stereos, cars, and vacations. Our newest model 270 Norwalk has a stronger press and a new cutter design, that grinds more effortlessly than before, causing even less oxidation. Your Norwalk is guaranteed for 12 years and is available in black, white, or a more durable woodgrain or stainless finish. **Compare the advantages of the Norwalk Juicer and Order Yours Today !**

Factory direct prices:
270-S Norwalk stainless ....$1995 _____
270 Norwalk woodgrain ....$1945 _____
270 Norwalk __ black or __ white ....$1895 _____

__ extra sets filter cloths at $15 __ extra sets filter bags at $16............... _____
California Residents **or** those taking delivery in Ca. add tax:
(270S - $139 270 Wood - $136   270 B or W - $132)................... _____

All Sales Are Final.   *Total* ......   _____

Payment options: **Cash** , Check, **Visa, M.C.**

Delivery Options :
1. **Pick-up** at Solana Beach Ca.
2. UPS to Continental U.S.A. -- **No Charge.**
(Allow 3-7 working days delivery)
3. Alaska, Hawaii, or **2 day air $50. 1 day air $100.**

4. OUTSIDE U.S.A. **270 or 270-S EXPORTED 110V or 220V.**
Freight charges & duty collected by Emery Air upon delivery.

To Order a Norwalk Juicer Call 1(800)405-8423
For other reasons or outside U.S.A. call (619)755-8423

Name:_____

Address: _____

_____

Zip:_____Phone # (____) _____

Norwalk Juicers
145 E. Cliff St. Solana Beach, CA. 92075
Office Hours and Demonstrations by Appointment Only

The Ecovortek unit

Victor Schauberger, an Austrian natural scientist and inventor studied water all his life. He said *"the mysteries of water are similar to those of blood in the human body. In nature, normal functions are fulfiled by water just as blood provides many important functions for mankind"*.

The Ecovortek unit is designed to put life back into water, and activated water enlivens the human being. Drinking and using water from an Ecovortek unit has many benefits:

- Descales kettles, baths and shower alcoves, making them easier to clean
- No running costs
- Maintenance free
- Users report an improvement in the feeling of well-being and aerobic fitness
- Softens water without using chemicals
- Reduces the use of detergents sand shampoo to achieve the same results.

All enquiries and orders:

The Water Shop
Water World
Shop 4A Western Roadway
Adelaide Central Market SA
Tel: (08) 8231 3311

Ecovortek Pty Ltd
PO Box 6142
Halifax Street
Adelaide SA 5000
Email: ecovortek@de-fontenay.com

JUICES

People always ask me "what type of juice do you drink?" The juice my family and I are currently taking is a combination of spinach, celery, parsley, cabbage and carrot. The next question I am asked is "in what quantities of each do you mix to make a juice?" My response to this is that it really depends on personal taste and it is best to experiment as I did until you come up with the best combination.

However my recipe for the juice is as follows.

COMBINATION VEGETABLE JUICE

2 large spinach leaves with spine cut out, cut into pieces
1 handfuls of cut up cabbage
2 celery sticks cut into pieces
1 medium carrot cut into pieces (peeled)
1 handful of parsley
1 handful of fennel leaf optional, it gives the juice a refreshing taste, very much like aniseed and fennel is very good for digestion.

Wash all vegetables and cut up into small pieces as it is easier to put through the juicer. The spinach tends to froth quite a lot so when juicing, start with half the spinach, celery, carrot, parsley and fennel. Then repeat. You will need to strain the juice through a sieve before drinking. This recipe is enough for one large glass or two small glasses.

BEETROOT AND APPLE

Another juice which our kids especially enjoy is beetroot and apple:

1 small beetroot scrubbed. Cut off top and bottom and quarter
3 medium sized granny smith apples scrubbed and quartered with
core cut out.
1 pea size piece of fresh ginger

This juice also will need to be filtered as the beetroot creates froth. This juice has a truly exotic taste. It is very refreshing and the kids love it! It can be watered down.

A juice we have in between our own juices is the Breuss juice, mentioned on page 132. The juice consists of beetroot, carrot, celeriac, potato and radish. It can be bought in 500ml bottles from health shops around Australia. The juice goes under the name of BIOTTA, distributed by Herbal Supplies Pty Ltd. Tel: (08) 8262 453.

BREUSS JUICE

You can alternatively make your own. The juice consists of:

300g beetroot, 100g carrots, 100g celeriac, 70g potato,
30g radish (chinese)

Once put through the juicer, this juice also needs to be filtered. For more information about the juice and its potential benefits, you can refer to the book "Cancer, Leukaemia The Breuss Cancer Cure" by Rudolph Breuss with Hilde Hemmes. Available at Health shops and Bookstores. *(For further details, refer to Book Reviews, page 230).*

Recommended reading for more information relating to a variety of juices used to help various ailments is "Fresh Vegetable and Fruit Juices" by Dr Norman Walker (ISBN 0-89019-06704).

COMPLIMENTARY THERAPEUTIC PROCEDURES

If you decide to take on the Gerson Therapy, then I applaud you. You have at least taken the initiative to try something completely natural. Wherever possible, try to keep in touch with a physician who is open-minded about what you are about to do. Some physicians know or have at least heard about the Gerson Therapy, and their assistance and guidance would be tremendous for you. Once again, I implore anyone interested, to read, "A CANCER THERAPY", by Max Gerson which will guide you through step by step and you will be able to read the results of fifty cured cases.

As I mentioned earlier, I will try to explain as best I can, my own experiences relating to the enemas and pain. Whilst I was on the full therapy I was fortunate enough to be under the care of a physician in Mexico, so any pain I felt, would soon be reported to my physician. I suffered little pain and I had several 'flare-ups'. Flare-ups are considered a form of healing reactions occurring within the body. On several occasions upon returning home, when I did experience such a flare-up, I would immediately administer a castor oil pack to the location of my pain, followed immediately by a coffee enema. The transition was instant. For your convenience, I have set out below extracts in part from the Gerson Primer and from taped lectures. It outlines in brief what to do when experiencing pain and different alternative pain relief methods.

Pain

Pain medications are often toxic and may interfere with the Gerson diet therapy. Whenever possible, use non-toxic methods to reduce and control pain. During reactions of 'flare ups', pain can be caused or worsened when substantial amounts of toxins are circulating throughout the blood system. They irritate the nerves in damaged and diseased areas of the body. By lowering toxic levels, this irritation and pain can be lessened. This is done by more frequent enemas. Research has shown that the body has its own natural pain killers. Most patients can testify to the fact that enemas relate directly to lowered pain levels.

Pain Triad

The triad should be used sparingly and should not exceed 6 dosages in a 24 hour period. The triad consists of 50mg niacin, 500mg ascorbic acid (Vitamin C) and a 300mg aspirin.

The Pain Triad becomes progressively more effective as the body undergoes detoxification. It can be used at bedtime to assist in going to sleep for those patients with substantial pain.

Castor Oil Pack

1. *Soak 3 pieces of white flannel with castor oil. Squeeze out excess.*
2. *Place flannel over affected area.*
3. *Place slightly larger sheet of plastic over the flannel.*
4. *Use medium temperature heating pad or hot water bottle over area. Don't let the pack get cold or uncomfortably hot.*
5. *Keep on 1/2 hour; apply every four hours. You can re-use the castor oil pack.*

This procedure is used during severe flare-ups involving liver pain, bile system spasms, or severe pain at other sites. It can also be used by arthritic patients over swollen painful joints. It is a bit messy when used over hands and feet, but effective.

Enemas

Intestinal spasms and cramping: These frequently painful symptoms are caused by strong irritation to the intestinal tract and lead to problems with the enemas. It becomes difficult to instill the full litre of coffee solution, difficult to hold the enema the full 12-15 minutes, or on the other hand, the enema becomes trapped and cannot be released. Following is a list of possible remedies which have proved useful to other patients:

1. CHECK THE ENEMA TECHNIQUE

Be sure that the tip of the enema tube is inserted five to six inches past the anal sphincter. There are nelaton tubes available from medical suppliers, that will attach to the end of most enema hoses. Do not try to force the tube into the colon. The temperature of the enema solution must be body temperature, 38°C . Don't raise the enema bucket too high. If the flow is too rapid it can set up counter-spasms. About 18-24 inches is the correct bucket height. Even at that height, spasms can occur. If so, immediately lower the bucket to allow the flow to back up a few inches into the tube to relieve the pressure. After 20-30 seconds, slowly start raising the bucket toward the original level. The flow can also be controlled by pinching the tube with your fingers or adjusting the plastic ring to a partially closed position. It may take some time to get the enema completely instilled, but this is acceptable.

2. HEAT OVER THE ABDOMEN

This can be applied by a heating pad. This has a calming effect on the irritated, hyperactive intestinal tract.

3. CAMOMILE TEA ENEMA

Use full strength and give just prior to the regularly scheduled coffee enema. Retain the tea enema for about five minutes. After release, immediately start the coffee enema. In severe problems, camomile concentrate can be added to all coffee enemas.

Recipe for a single camomile enema
4 tablespoons camomile flowers, dried and organic
1 litre of water
Boil 5 minutes and simmer for 10 minutes. Strain. Use cooled to body temperature.

Recipe for camomile concentrate (4 enemas)
1 cup camomile flowers dried.
2 cups water

Simmer 30 minutes in covered saucepan. Strain and press camomile flowers to extrude fluid. If some has boiled away, add distilled water to make 0.5 litre. Keep in covered glass bottle no longer than 3 days. To use, pour 125ml concentrate into enema bucket and fill with distilled water.

4. ADD POTASSIUM COMPOUND

Potassium compound solution added to the enema helps relieve spasms by supplying potassium to the depleted intestinal tract. It can also help to promote bile flow when given rectally. This solution is the same as that used in the juices. The dosage is two tablespoons in each enema. Procedure should be discontinued after 10 days to 2 weeks.

5. LOWER THE DOSAGE

This can be accomplished by either using less coffee concentrate in each enema or by using only part of a prepared enema. Consult with a physician if possible.

6. BACK-TO-BASICS ENEMAS

When the first enema is 'clutched' and the abdomen congested, a second enema may be taken 'back to back' with the first. Potassium compound solution may be added to the second enema to promote effectiveness. Another potentially valuable aid is hydrogen peroxide (1-2 tsp: 3%) added to the second enema. Camomile concentrate may be added to counter the irritating effects of either peroxide or potassium taken by rectum.

Caution: If you run into chronic problems, please do not resort to a long series of consecutive enemas (use no more than 3 back to back). At least four hours must be allowed between back to back enemas in most cases. *Please be in touch with your physician.*

Castor oil enemas may also be used in some cases if a back to back enema is also 'clutched'. *Castor Oil enemas are extremely pushy and should be used cautiously — generally only one in a 24 hour period. Consult your physician.* (For Castor Oil Enema preparation, see page 108).

FLARE-UPS AND REACTIONS

Notes from a lecture by Dr Dan Rogers, MD.

Definition of Flare-Up/Reaction: The response elicited the immune system in particular and the body in general by an intensification of the detoxification process.

Causes: The causes can be many — the body's attempt to rid itself of dead and diseased tissue and cells, eliminate toxins of all types, and rebuild healthy cells and tissues.

Flare-ups may include any of the following symptoms:

1. *Flu-like symptoms:* Including general aches and pains, sore muscles and joints, that 'achey all-over feeling',

fairly common in most patients. Duration is usually 24-48 hours. Usually self-limited.

Rx: (Remedy) Treat symptomatically including clay/castor oil packs, pain triad and bed rest.

2. **Nausea:** May be intense, lasting for several days. Usually self-limited.

Rx: Treat symptomatically. Increase intake of peppermint tea and oatmeal. May need to decrease oral solid intake or exchange it for raw grated apples, applesauce, raw grated carrots, mashed banana, watermelon etc. Also change juice composition by adding up to 50% gruel per juice. May give gruel straight.*(refer page 96)*

3. **Vomiting:** Does not occur in most cases. If it does occur it usually lasts 24 hours or less. Some cases can be intense and of longer duration requiring definitive treatment, especially when complicated by other body fluid loss such as diarrhoea, or in a patient with reduced body mass (ie. child cachexia: a chronic state of malnutrition, etc.)

Rx: Increase peppermint tea intake to as much as 3 litres or more and substitute oatmeal for regular meals when needed. May need to decrease oral solid intake or exchange it for raw grated vegetables and fruit. Also exchange juice composition by adding up to 50% gruel per juice. May also give gruel straight. Juices not taken orally can be given rectally as a retention enema. If vomiting lasts longer than 24 hours, then see GP.

4. **Diarrhoea:** Frequent passage of unformed, watery bowel movements. If it occurs it is usually self-limiting lasting 24-48 hours. If it persists any longer, definitive treatment may be required, especially when complicated by other body fluid loss and it would be wise to consult with your GP.

   Rx: Consult with your GP.

5. **Pain:** May be prodromal (ie. signalling a flare-up) starting as much as 48-72 hours prior to reaction. Usually self-limiting. Duration up to 72 hours post reaction. May require definitive Rx.

   Rx: Treat symptomatically. Use increased enemas, clay/castor oil packs and pain triad as first treatment of choice. Amigadalina is a good Rx alternative especially with bony metastases (the spreading of a disease from one organ to another). *(refer to pages 94, 95, 105, 108, 242)*

6. **Chills and Fever:** May last 24-48 hours, usually self-limited. For the most part should be treated with physical means. Area of precaution include high fevers (greater than 39°C) for a period greater than 2 hours, and patients with reduced body mass (ie. child, cachexia, etc.).

   Rx: For chills use physical means as first treatment of choice. Put the patient to bed, warm them with blankets, pyjamas, etc. May also enjoy warm bath, hot tea, etc. Bed rest is advisable. For fever, also use physical means as first treatment of choice. Reduce amount of constrictive clothing, remove most blankets, but maintain normal environmental temperatures. Use vinegar/alcohol rub down, cool water rub down, damp cloth on neck/forehead, etc. Bed rest is advisable. If the patient's temperature continues to rise, cool tea/coffee/water enemas may be needed. Also, cool baths with up to full body immersion may be used. If fever is still rising, the pain triad, with emphasis on aspirin, may be employed. Try to avoid the use of any stronger anti-fever agents, except for very unusual circumstances. Careful monitoring of the patient is ESSENTIAL if physical means are to be successful in controlling fever, especially if body temperature remains at 37°C or more. If physical means plus aspirin and careful monitoring do not control fever at a manageable level, definitive treatment must be employed.

7. **Foul smells:** This general category includes breath, body odour, smelly enemas, etc. At least one of these symptoms is fairly common in patients during their first reactions. They are self-limiting lasting the duration of the reaction, and up to 48 hours post reaction. No special precautions need to be taken, except for the comfort of the patient and any visitors.

Rx: Brush teeth several times per day. Eat garlic. Drink extra juice/tea.

Body Odour: Bathe and change clothes often. Vinegar/alcohol rubdown. Drink extra juice/tea.

Enema odour: Increase number of enemas including castor oil (*check with your physician*). Instruct everyone to leave the room at enema time and open the bathroom windows, even in the winter. May need to repaint the room.

8. **Depression:** This symptom is very common to many patients, especially during the first several reactions. It is due in part to the increase of toxins, released into the blood, on the brain and its functions. It may be a prodromal sign of an upcoming reaction, occurring as much as 72 hours before the reaction starts. It worsens as the reaction occurs, and may last 72 hours following the flare-up. It is usually self-limiting. The patient especially needs as much extra 'tender loving care' (TLC) as possible at this time.

   Rx: Treat symptomatically. Lots of support, TLC, encouragement, companion and family support are especially critical here.

9. **Jaundice/Ictericia:** Duration usually limited to 48 hours, post flare-up.

   Rx: No definitive treatment. Increase juices and enemas.

Note: Remember flare-ups can consist of one or more of the above symptoms, and perhaps all of them.

Again I stress to consult with a physician where possible to help you along and give you guidance should you be concerned about any one matter.

Another extract from the Gerson Primer, is the subject on cosmetics, teeth, sunscreen, colds and flu, exercise and protein.

COSMETICS

All substances which go on the skin at best clog pores and keep the skin from breathing and eliminating toxins. At worst, these materials are absorbed into the blood stream and damage the patient. While on the intensive therapy, the patient should refrain from using ANY skin lotions, creams, and ointments whatsoever. Especially, women need to refrain from using lipstick which is regularly licked off the lips and therefore ingested. Sometimes, women complain that their lips are dry or raw if they do not use lipstick. This is often due to the lipstick. If the patient refrains from its use for a few days, uses a little Vaseline, the lips 'heal' and will feel normal.

We feel very strongly about any underarm anti-perspirant or deodorant. ALL these are harmful, even if purchased in a 'health food store'. Many contain aluminium, and other chemicals which should never be applied to underarms.

They not only block the lymphatics but are absorbed and toxic. The passages should be clear and open for elimination of toxic perspiration. If sweat is smelly, wash frequently and keep the lymph passages OPEN. To block them is to force the toxic materials back into the lymph passages to cause new harm. Once the body is well detoxified, it will not have any unpleasant smell.

Nail polish keeps the nails from breathing. Do not use it while on the Gerson Therapy; nor any artificial nails.

We need not mention permanents or hair dyes, since these are mentioned on the list of FORBIDDEN ITEMS in A Cancer Therapy *(page 210)*. However, hair sprays, lacquers with acetone solvents, are also very harmful and have to be avoided. On the therapy, your hair will become healthier and have natural 'body'. You will not need some of the toxic cosmetics.

TEETH

A very important consideration for success on the Gerson Therapy is the need to clear any possible dental root abscess. Sometimes, these abscesses cause no symptoms and the patient is not aware of them. Also, some patients are overly concerned about X-rays, to the point that they even refuse the small amount of radiation used to diagnose possible dental problems. That is a mistake. The amount of radiation is not harmful; but the possible existence of dental root canal infections or abscesses will negate the effectiveness of the Gerson Therapy. Sometimes seriously damaged or infected teeth have to be removed in order to eliminate the constant 're-infection' caused by these toxins in the mouth. Please check your teeth and make sure that there are no dental problems as you start on the Therapy.

Another possible dental problem is mercury. Most people are now aware that the so-called 'silver amalgam' fillings contain about 51% mercury. This is a highly toxic heavy metal which affects not only the nervous system but can cause untold problems and can counteract the healing effect of the Gerson

Therapy. There are now techniques available for removing these amalgam fillings correctly (*see Dr Hal Huggins, "IT'S ALL IN YOUR HEAD"*). However, no matter how carefully the fillings are removed, some of the mercury is activated and re-enters the system. This causes a temporary mercury poisoning, which is fairly easily overcome by the Gerson Therapy. However, it is unwise to subject the seriously or terminally ill patient, just starting the Gerson Therapy, to this additional poisoning. We therefore suggest that the patient waits at least 6-12 months until he is much improved before considering the removal of the offending fillings. Many dentists refuse to do this work. Refer to the above book, to Dr Huggin's office in Colorado Springs, and he will give you names in your area of dentists who will do the work. Silver amalgam fillings can be replaced with various plastic materials which are now available. Gold fillings are also acceptable; however occasionally dentists have placed gold crowns on top of silver amalgam fillings in the same tooth. This is highly damaging.

In one respect, your dentist could cause you considerable trouble namely if he recommends for you to brush your teeth with baking soda. 'Soda' is sodium. It is very easily absorbed through the mucus membranes in the mouth and quickly enters the blood stream. We have had one patient who came to us with a colon cancer. On the therapy, after about 10 months, she was completely cleared of cancer. She continued the therapy, faithfully, as she had been instructed. Nevertheless, after another 6 months or so, she had a new malignant lesion in her colon.

When we returned to CHIPSA hospital, upon intensive questioning, it turned out that her dentist had suggested that she brush her teeth with baking soda. She did — and her tumour returned. When she was told to stop this practice, she again healed.

We need to warn patients not to follow such dentists' instructions. Also, please note that Dr Gerson's book (*page 210*), states on the list of "FORBIDDEN ITEMS" not to use baking soda also for gargling, etc. The above patient did not remember or check on this before following her dentist's instructions. Please also note that MANY brands of toothpaste presently contain baking soda — since dentists recommend it. Please do not use such toothpastes. (non flouride toothpastes are available from most health stores)

SUNSCREEN

Dr Gerson did not want patients to be exposed to sun, nor to sunbathe. During the last few years, it has become fashionable to recommend 'sunscreen' because many doctors claim that sunlight can cause skin cancer. Dr Gerson's reason for recommending to avoid sunlight is that it is radiation, it is wearying and irritating, so the patient must avoid it., sunscreen is not the answer. On the contrary, the latest information has it that the sunscreen which people are supposed to use and put on their children's skin becomes a carcinogen (cancer causing agent) when exposed to the sun! If you are going out, wear a long-sleeved shirt, preferably white cotton, or a blouse. Use a hat with a wide brim or visor to protect your face. You need not stay indoors altogether when the weather is sunny. Just don't expose yourself without clothes, to 'sunbathe'. It is always suggested that you take in fresh air, IN THE SHADE, under a tree or umbrella. If you are using the sun 'to warm you', rather use extra covers, sweaters, coats or blankets, but stay in the shade.

COLDS AND FLU

There is presently in the general population quite a serious problem consisting of depressed immune systems. There is a constant increase in infections which were virtually unknown a decade ago: AIDS, 'chronic fatigue syndrome' (Epstein-Barr), genital herpes, hepatitis of all kinds and candida (yeast infections). Other infectious diseases which seemed to have almost disappeared, such as tuberculosis, and even syphilis, are making a threatening comeback.

It has to be assumed that the poor general nutrition, together with excess consumption of fats, proteins and salt, cause these health problems. Obviously, patients suffering from cancer also have a weakened immune system — since a fully functioning immune response is capable of protecting the body from ever developing cancer. So, we know that in all cancer patients, we have a problem if they 'catch' cold or develop a flu. Even after a few months on the Gerson Therapy, which among other things restores the immune system, the former cancer patient does not yet have a good defence against cold and flu viruses. For that reason, much care has to be taken to protect the recovering patient from visitors, kids or other household members who have colds. They should be completely segregated. Friends of visitors with colds would either be requested not to visit, or, if they have come into the house, the patient should quietly (even unsociably!) disappear behind his/her bedroom door.

If a recovering patient does develop a cold or flu, at the very first signs, he should take penicillin (other antibiotics if he is allergic to penicillin) together with the 'triad', at least once every 6 hours for as long as symptoms are present, plus one day. It is also wise to gargle with camomile tea in which you use 1.5ml of a 3% solution of hydrogen peroxide, at least three times a day. A very warm bath with at least 2.5L of 3% hydrogen peroxide twice a day is extremely helpful. Be sure that the patient is not chilled upon leaving the bath and immediately goes into a warm bed. A cold should be treated with great respect since it can cause recurrence of tumours.

EXERCISE

Dr Gerson felt very strongly that a cancer patient just starting on the Therapy, urgently needs rest. He even had patients who were not particularly debilitated, stay in bed for a full six weeks! The Gerson Therapy also will speed up the metabolism which required energy. This energy requirement often causes patients starting the treatment to be tired. This is an urgent message of the body to rest! Do not force exercise when you are tired, it will not 'build you up' at all, on the contrary, it will slow down or stop healing if you waste your energy.

Early on in the treatment, it is good practice to do some trampolining. A little 'rebounder' is quite inexpensive, and can be very helpful. In the beginning, use it only by lifting your heel and bending your knees — don't jump. Also, it is best to use it for only 30 seconds at a time, but several times a day — as often as 5-6 times. This very mild exercise stimulates lymphatic circulation and also helps to overcome pain, especially bone pain. But again, don't overdo it or exhaust yourself!

When patients first return home, they usually feel much better, but not yet strong. It is extremely important that they do not immediately jump into their jobs or housework — since the Therapy with all the foods and juices is very work intensive. The patient needs continued rest and HELP. Usually, after about three months, energy comes back again. That, too, could be a period of danger: when the patient is recovering and feels energy coming back, he/she may well start into strenuous activities — overexerting himself, and stopping the healing. DO NO OVERDO. As energy returns, you can start on some very mild 'exercise': a five-minute walk! (Not in extreme heat or cold). This can soon be extended to 8-10 minutes — but, if the patient is very tired, STOP IT, and go back to the last amount of walking that didn't exhaust you. Increase the time for a walk very slowly if you can easily handle it. More strenuous exercise (tennis, squash) must be avoided for a year or so. Swimming is a problem, all chlorinated pools must be completely avoided, ocean water is too salty for the patient. So what remains? A clean mountain stream or lake. 'Clean' means that there are no factories above the place where you swim, which drain chemicals into the water. And, of course, the weather must be mild or warm, so the patient is not chilled. One of our recovered breast cancer patients in Carmel, California, after some 4 years on the Therapy and total recovery, has won several tennis tournaments. Just be patient and heal first!

PROTEINS

After approximately 6-10 weeks on the Therapy, your doctor will order you to start on some NON-FAT, UNSALTED, UN FLAVOURED, MODIFIED milk proteins. This does NOT mean LOW FAT (yoghurt or cottage cheese). In Dr Gerson's book, you will find that he ordered for the patient to take buttermilk and/or 'pot-cheese'. We have to be very careful with these items nowadays. Buttermilk comes in two forms:'churned' and 'cultured'. The churned type is good and acceptable — but it is almost never available anymore. If you have a dairy farmer in your neighbourhood who will churn some sour cream to make his own butter, and let you have the buttermilk — that would be great. But, otherwise, don't bother looking for it. The 'Cultured' type is completely forbidden. It is usually made of left-over unsaleable milk, treated with thickening agents; flavoured AND SALTED!

The next problem is 'Pot Cheese'. In Dr Gerson's day, this meant non-fat, unsalted cottage cheese which he approved of. Today, this is no longer available. All cottage cheese is creamed and salted; the 'Low-Fat' type is usually 2% butterfat (much too much) and is also salted. Sometimes, you can obtain so-called baker's cheese, which is supposed to be used in baking and is not supposed to contain cream or salt. This is all right to use; however, it is tasteless. So you have to add non-fat, unflavoured yoghurt to it, whip it up with onion, garlic, chives, etc. and make it into a delicious spread. Be sure that the cheese is free of cream and salt. One patient was using a cottage cheese, made by a farmer using his own 'cottage industry' recipe, which was simple hard cheese, with about 40% butterfat and salt! Of course, her tumours recurred...

Another problem is yoghurt. It has to be non-fat and unflavoured. Some patients are trying their best to do right, and look for raw, unpasteurized milk yoghurt. BE CAREFUL. You will possibly find raw goat's milk yoghurt, and think you have it made. NOT SO. Goat's milk is by nature homogenised, and it is difficult to remove the cream — so it is left full fat. We lost one patient because the care-giver was not aware of the danger of raw goat's milk yoghurt.

You can also be confused by labels; one set of information on your yoghurt container will be 'Ingredients'. Obviously, this should only include non-fat milk and cultures. The other information on your container will be 'analysis of content'. I have had many calls from patients saying that yoghurt contains sodium. Of course, all milk contains a certain amount of natural sodium — don't worry about it. The problem is only caused by any addition of salt, which will show in the 'Ingredients'.

Very rarely, a patient is lactose intolerant and cannot handle any milk products. Your doctor may advise you to take spirulina, blue-green magma, or bee-pollen. This too, can sometimes cause allergic reactions. If you are trying it, use just a few grains at first, and add a few at a time before reaching your prescribed amount. *If it causes you any allergic reaction, don't use it.*

The above information is a very good guide for anyone undertaking the Gerson Therapy and again, where possible consultation from a physician would be an extreme help.

ADJUVANT THERAPIES

The following adjuvant therapies should not be taken on their own, but as the name suggests, should be taken as part of an existing nutritional therapy.

OXYGEN THERAPY

Studies have shown that oxygen therapies produce desirable results in cancer treatment, as most pathogenic organisms require low oxygen levels for their survival. Boosting oxygen levels revitalises normal cells whilst killing some viruses and pathogens. Two types of oxygen therapies I used were Ozone (O_3) and Hydrogen Peroxide (H_2O_2) therapies. Hydrogen Peroxide is a by-product of Ozone. Ozone is easily produced via a Ozone generator which can be ordered within Australia (*see health magazines or retail outlets*). Hydrogen Peroxide is readily available from pharmacies and supermarkets in liquid form in either 3%, or 6% solution. Hydrogen Peroxide is exceptional in cases of mouth ulcers, sore throat and as a general disinfectant. I gargle with approximately 1ml of Hydrogen Peroxide in a 250ml glass of water.

Ozone was administered rectally three times a day at a dose of approximately 30°C. I was required to lay down for half an hour after administration. Hydrogen Peroxide is produced when ozone contacts water. It can be taken orally, absorbed through the skin by bathing in a diluted solution, or intravenously. *(For more information, refer to Book Reviews, page 228).*

ESSIAC TEA (PAU D'ARCO OR TAHEBO TEA)

Made up of various herb combinations which have been used by native American Indians, these teas have been shown to have anti-cancer and immune enhancing properties. *(Refer to Book Reviews — The Essiac Report, page 229)*

VITAMIN C

After reading the book Cancer and Vitamin C *(refer to Book Reviews, page 215)*, I decided that this was an additional therapy that not only I, but also my entire family could benefit from. The results were immediate.

It can be used orally, intravenously and rectally. One protocol uses Laetrile *(see below)* and Vitamin C for the treatment of patients that have previously had chemotherapy.

AMYGDALINE / LAETRILE

This is the purified form of amygdalin which is also known as Vitamin B-17, which occurs naturally in the kernels of apricots and in some other foods. Laetrile is a cyanogenic glycoside (containing cyanide). It is believed that laetrile is non-toxic and has anti-cancer properties. It also has been used for pain relief.

POLARISING TREATMENT

The polarising treatment is a solution consisting of potassium chloride and insulin in glucose solution which is given intravenously. It is used over a two to three day period, and in some cases, a thirty day period. This treatment stimulates healing, restoration of potassium to its proper level within the cells, production of free energy through oxidative phosphorylation, lowering of intracellular acidoses, recycling of fatty acids and other lipids and stimulation of protein synthesis.

Polarising treatment promotes healing in the diseased heart, and in tissues damaged by cancer and other degenerative disease. Polarizing solution serves as a non-toxic but potent pain relief. Dramatic reductions in pain levels, during and following solution application, is noticed. Excess fluids in feet, ankles, abdomen face, etc., is rapidly re absorbed and released from the body.

HYPERBARIC OXYGEN (HBO) THERAPY

This therapy is used specifically for increasing oxygen levels of the body in general and in tumour tissue in particular.

HYDROTHERAPY

This treatment requires the patient be immersed in a bathtub containing water above body temperature. This will cause a mild induced fever. When laetrile has already been injected prior to the bath, the temperature at the tumour site is further increased which gives the body an even better opportunity to destroy the tumour tissue. Normal healthy body tissue can easily withstand temperatures up to 38°C; however tumour tissue cannot.

CARTILAGE

This is available in two forms, either bovine or shark. Very recent experiments with cartilage, have shown beneficial effects for cancer patients. There are various methods of application, including rectal implant.

WOBE MUGOS

These are highly concentrated pancreatic enzymes. These help to dissolve and digest tumour tissue. These are not available in Australia and I had to specifically request them on the medical form when placing an order. The price is approximately US$200 per pack of 100 tablets.

Complimentary Supplements

FOR CHEMOTHERAPY, RADIOTHERAPY, SURGERY AND HORMONAL TREATMENT

Time and time again, people have come to me for advice on what to do and what to take to help boost their immune system whilst undergoing chemotherapy, radiotherapy, surgery or hormonal treatment.

From my observations of others, I have found that the following supplements have assisted significantly in reducing undesirable side effects.

Large doses of Vitamin A, B-Complex, C, Zinc, Selenium, B12, Niacin, Digestive Enzymes, Acidophilus capsules or powder combined with a diet similar to that of Gerson will assist the body's immune system.

It is my recommendation to seek advice from a competent Naturopath or Holistic Practitioner for individual requirements.

PRAYER

Last but by far not the least is prayer. Praying for help and healing in time of illness is a common practice amongst most western cultures. Praying to the Judeo-Christian God for the benefit of others — intercessory prayer — is widely accepted and practised. Nevertheless, the medical literature rarely examines whether or not intercessory prayer is therapeutically effective.

Studies done on patients who received intercessory prayer from several Protestant churches and the Roman Catholic church, upon entering hospital with cardiac and non cardiac (such as pneu-monia or diabetes) conditions, showed fewer life threatening events and complications during their stay in the coronary care unit, than the patients who did not receive prayer. Patients who received intercessory prayer were unaware of the fact.

Prayer is a great healer, so I encourage you to pray to whomever your god is.

COMPLIMENTARY
THERAPIES

It seems that the more time goes by, the more I come into contact with people and information relating to alternative therapies. I have researched many of these therapies and applied them to myself and my family where and when possible.

I would like to outline some of these therapies as they would be beneficial not only to the cancer patient but also to every person striving for a healthier life.

Konstantin P. Buteiko, MD, PhD (b.1923)

Assigned as a medical student to monitor dying patients' breathing, Buteiko found that the sicker they grew, the deeper they breathed. He learned to predict the day and even the hour of death.

Knowing that no one would pay heed to his work without laboratory studies, he established a series of functional diagnostics laboratories. In 1958-59, he showed the USSR Academy of Science a linear relationship between the depth of breathing, the content of CO_2 in the body, vessel spasming and degrees of illness. By the end of 1966 he and his students had treated more than 1,000 patients including themselves for asthma, hypertension or heart pain. All of them substantially recovered, some from 20 or more conditions none had been helped by allopathic treatments.

Like every revolutionary new medical technique, Buteiko's treatment was long rejected and he suffered personal abuse. One laboratory after another was destroyed or disbanded, yet he and his students pushed on; his method has been Russian government approved since 1983. It has been practiced ever since with an high degree of success throughout Russia, and more recently in Australia.

Source: Townsend Letter for Doctors & Patients, January 1998

BUTEIKO METHOD OF BREATHING

Working for several years in the Siberian Branch of the USSR Academy of Sciences on the problems of breathing and blood circulation, Dr Buteiko found out that the cause of the most wide-spread diseases was deep breathing (alveolar hyper-ventilation). The very deep breathing, which was considered to be a remedy for many diseases, proved to be their cause.

With the help of a unique equipment complex, a mathematical dependence of pathogenic processes from the depth of breathing was proved and the harm of deep breathing through the loss of carbon dioxide in lungs, blood, and organism cells was explained. The norm of carbon dioxide quantity was found out as well as mathematical formulas of the state of health.

Deviation from this norm with absolute exactness allowed to foresee the emergence of the illness. The laws of health and diseases were opened and they were proved by mathematical calculations.

As it was found out, various diseases, such as BRONCHIAL ASTHMA, ALLERGIES, HYPERTENSION, GASTRITIS, EXZEMA etc., are the consequences of one illness — DEEP BREATHING and have one cause — DEEP BREATHING. Moreover, the BLOCKING OF NOSE, ASTHMATIC FIT — all this is just a way of organism defence from constant deep breathing and all these symptoms disappear while the patient gets rid of deep breathing. EASY FATIGUABILITY, LOW EFFICIENCY — these are also deep breathing symptoms.

On the basis of his discovery, Dr Buteiko worked out a most effective non-medicinal method of treatment, which allows to do away with the symptoms mentioned and to get rid of the disease without any medicine.

The essence of the Buteiko method concerns the gradual reduction of the depth of breathing to the 'norm' by way of rational, persistent and constant relaxation of breathing muscles with the obligatory measurements of carbon dioxide in the lungs.

ASTHMA AND BUTEIKO

"Asthma is not a disease", Buteiko asserted, but one of the body's defensive mechanisms against hyperventilation. He discovered that the average person with asthma breathes three to twelve times the recommended amount. The body slowly increases bronchospasm and mucous production — its defenses against overbreathing. Bronchodilator medications ease the tightness experienced during an asthma attack, overriding the defensive mechanism — and so gradually the condition worsens.

It is widely acknowledged that asthmatics benefit from swimming yet other forms of exercise trigger 'exercise induced asthma'. The secret: swimmers gradually release their breath while swimming with their face under water, then turn the head and inhale quickly. There isn't time to overbreathe.

Principles of the Buteiko Method

WHAT IS NORMAL BREATHING?

At rest we should breathe about 4–6 litres of air per minute. We should breathe mainly with our diaphragm.

WHAT IS HYPERVENTILATION?

Hyperventilation is defined as ventilation in excess of metabolic requirements. HV is breathing more than 6 litres per minute at rest.

WHY IS IT IMPORTANT TO BREATHE CORRECTLY?

The gas mix in the air we breathe, is different to the gas mix we need to maintain in our lungs and body. The gas mix in the air contains about 21% O_2 (oxygen) — 0.03% CO_2 (carbon dioxide) compared to the gas mix in our lungs, which is required to contain 14% O_2 — 5% (6.5%) CO_2.

In the external air there are only traces of CO_2, therefore we have to produce the CO_2 required to create the correct gas balance in our lungs and body through metabolic processes.

HYPERVENTILATION, WHAT HAPPENS?

If we breathe too much, we exhale more CO_2 than we produce, which means we lose CO_2. (Average asthmatics are known to over-breathe 2x–3x the recommended amount).

Prolonged sleep, especially on the back or with the mouth open, or both (as is common among asthmatics), encourages hyperventilation. One should sleep on one side rather than the back. A more reliable way to minimize mouth breathing in sleep is to tape the mouth shut.

WHAT IS THE ROLE OF CO_2 IN OUR BODY?

1. CO_2 is our body's own natural bronchodilator, blood vessel dilator and smooth muscle dilator.

2. CO_2 is the body's most important buffer in the regulation of the body's acid/alkaline balance. Low levels of CO_2 may lead to respiratory alkalosis. The alkaline shifts interfere with metabolic processes and cause a weakening in the immune system, which can manifest in allergies, susceptibility to colds, flus and viruses, infections, excessive growth in bone tissue and may lead to the development of tumours.

3. Lowered levels of CO_2 strengthens the bond between haemoglobin and O_2 molecules, therefore making it difficult

for sufficient oxygenation of the tissues of the brain and other vital organs. Lowered levels of O_2 produce oxygen starvation of the tissue cells (hyposia).

4. O_2 starvation causes a false feeling of insufficiency of air, shortness of breath — this prompts the patient to breathe deeper. But the deeper the breathing the greater the O_2 starvation becomes and the vicious circle is completed.

WHAT IS A DEFENCE MECHANISM?

If CO_2 levels in the body fall below 3% the whole organism dies. Therefore the body tries to guard against excessive loss of CO_2. Once CO_2 levels have reached a point that is considered intolerable by the organism, the body creates a defence reaction, that manifests in — constriction of the pathways which serve CO_2 elimination (blocked nose, bronchospasm, mucus, polyp growth, spasm of arterial vessels, smooth muscles of intestine, biliary ducts, etc.) aimed at preventing further loss of CO_2 as well as attempting to raise CO_2 levels. Because the body uses the same channels for O_2 provision, these spasms create a shortage of O_2 supply to the brain, heart etc., which increases the O_2 starvation in the organism. Thus there is a very strict physiological law: *The greater the overbreathing, the less O_2 reaches the body's cells.*

THE REAL DISEASE

Dr Buteiko states, that the real disease behind Asthma, Allergies, Emphysema, Sleep apnoea, Sinus, etc., is:

Hyperventilation Syndrome or 'disease of deep breathing', resulting in the loss of CO_2 and consequent metabolic disturbances in the body. He further declares that Asthma, Allergies etc., are merely symptoms of Hyperventilation.

THE AIM OF THE BUTEIKO METHOD

The Buteiko Method aims at normalising the breathing rate and depth and therefore CO_2 levels (as well as removing the cause of hyperventilation), so that metabolic processes can be restored and healing can occur. As a result symptoms of hyperventilation subside in most cases completely.

I have applied the Buteiko Method of Breathing to myself and have found a remarkable difference to my health, in particular in the assistance of removal of mucus congestion in my chest and an improvement in my digestion. Also by taping the mouth shut, it eliminates snoring.

To learn more about the Buteiko method, you can attend a course as I did. Listed below are contact names in each state:

Adelaide, Perth   Carola Maier (08) 8398 2039
Northern Territory

Adelaide   Florian Maier (08) 8398 3883
*   Gesse Sleeman (08) 8398 2039*

Sydney   Greg Parnell (02) 9583 1212 (& NSW Country)
*   Rosalba Courtney-Belford (02) 9918 7422*

Brisbane	Patric Heineman (07) 3397 3832
	Lola Motina (07) 3892 7917
Townsville	James Hooper (0747) 255 160
Melbourne	Jeffrey Richards (03) 9532 5533
	Linda House (03) 9727 1105
Hobart	John Micheson (0362) 236 272

Recommended reading about the Buteiko Method of breathing is "Freedom From Asthma" by Alexander Stalatski (ISBN 1-085626-268-5).

Rudolph Breuss and his Vegetable Juice Diet

Rudolph Breuss, an Austrian, was born in 1899. He was in his forties when he began his career as a healing practitioner. During his earlier years he worked as an electrical engineer with most of his time spent in hospitals.

Observing first hand the illness of others during his working hours, coupled with his own health problems, he began to investigate alternative methods from those employed by orthodox medicine in the hospital.

It was a simple German book which captured his attention and which would direct his work for the rest of his life. Written over four hundred years earlier, the book explained in depth the value and use of fruit and vegetable juices.

For some time he experimented on himself to find the right mixture and balance of juices to serve the purpose of providing just sufficient nourishment to keep a person alive over a period long enough to clear the problem, particularly cancer.

His hypothesis was simple. Too simple to orthodox medical thinking. But during the 30 or more years he was in practice and some ten years after, until his death in 1991, the diet was to prove itself over and over again in so many cases. In fact, up until 1990, approximately 45,000 cancer patients and patients of seemingly incurable diseases, have recovered.

Rudolph Breuss maintained that cancer, wherever it occurs in the body, feeds and grows from protein. He therefore deduced that if one fasted for what has now been confirmed to be an ideal period of six weeks, during which various herb teas would be taken to detoxify, cleanse and eliminate, the cancer would starve and be absorbed and subsequently pass out of the body by one means or another.

What he sought was a selection of vegetable juices which would provide just enough nourishment to meet the basic requirements of the body during the six week period, but for all intents and purposes no protein, nor indeed the many and varied congesting foods which make up the normal diet.

The ultimate result was a mixture of organically grown vegetable juices comprising carrot, beetroot, continental radish celeriac, and potato. Not only was he meticulous in his instructions for making particular herb teas, but also with the vegetable juices. Each one had to be a specific quantity in order to get the right balance. In the early days he prepared the juices himself, then his patients made their own. To obtain all the vegetables from organic sources, even on the Continent, proved difficult, and such was the success of his treatment that the demand necessitated a more businesslike attitude to the problem.

Rudolph Breuss approached the Biotta company in Tagerwilen whom he gave the formula to make up the juice exactly as he wanted it, using tried and tested methods of preserving that life force in the juices which makes all Biotta juices so beneficial.

Breuss then tried out the results on a number of patients to ensure it was as effective as freshly expressing it, using a home juicer. It was. This was the breakthrough he needed, thus making it possible for people all over the world to use his system when suffering from cancer and other serious diseases.

The Biotta juices are now available in Australia in health shops. "Cancer Leukemia — The Breuss Cancer Cure" by Rudolph Breuss with Hilde Hemmes (ISBN 0-6-46-34773-X) is available in selected health shops and bookstores.

EDTA Chelation Therapy

WHAT IS CHELATION THERAPY?

Chelation therapy is the process whereby unwanted and potentially harmful metals are removed from the arteries, small blood vessels and body cells by slow intravenous infusion.

WHY DOES IT HELP HEART DISEASE?

EDTA binds to toxic metals such as lead, mercury, cadmium and aluminium and removes them in the urine. These toxic elements speed up the damage to our blood vessel linings caused by oxidised cholesterol. When nutrients called antioxidants are provided at the same time as the EDTA, natural healing proceeds faster than the damage by the cholesterol. This slowly removes the plaque that is blocking the blood vessels so that blood flow is improved. In addition, magnesium added to the solution dilates the blood vessels.

HOW EFFECTIVE IS IT?

More than 75 percent of patients treated have shown significant improvement from chelation therapy. More than 90 percent of patients receiving 35 or more treatments have benefited when they have also corrected dietary, exercise and smoking habits.

HOW IS IT DONE?

A course of treatment consists of 20-30 treatments in which EDTA and minerals and vitamins are infused into a vein of the arm over three hours while you sit in a recliner chair and doze or read.

WHAT DOES IT COST?

A course of treatment for a patient with advanced hardening of the arteries generally costs $2,000 to $3,000 for 20 to 30 treatments. For pensioners there is an 8% discount. Because there is no patent on EDTA there is no drug company promoting research and so it is not recognised by many cardiologists or the Australian Government as a useful treatment for atherosclerosis. This means that Medicare benefits are not payable for chelation therapy or for consultations related to it.

One patient said "It's less than a years Private Health Insurance and some years I don't get anything back. I'm getting a lot of benefit from this".

Chelation Treatment could save 'millions' of Heart Bypass Costs.

New Zealand MP Graeme Lee had Chelation in 1996 and attributes his excellent health and high energy to it. He remains extremely grateful for the bypass he had five years ago but has learnt about chelation since then and says "Chelation costs less than 1/10 of the cost of a heart bypass. Numerous patients have been taken off waiting lists for heart bypass surgery after having had Chelation and been retested by their cardiologists. This means that millions of dollars could be saved from the current bypass costs of NZ$M40-60 per year and waiting lists reduced."

An example of leg pain: One woman was unable to walk more than a few yards without suffering extreme pain in her right calf. After Chelation she has been able to travel to the UK and Bali on her own and has even been ballroom dancing. Occasionally when walking a long distance she has a slight pain, but if she stops for a minute it soon goes. The pulse in her leg was very slow and faint, but now it is quite healthy.

Chelation therapy produces a profoundly beneficial effect by excreting toxic metals and improving blood flow which in turn helps to regenerate many of our cellular life support systems.

CHELATION therapy has been proved by research to help in the following health problems:
- Arteriosclerosis (atherosclerosis)
- Angina
- High blood pressure
- High cholesterol
- Poor circulation (cold hands and feet)
- Leg ulceration and gangrene
- Intermittent claudication (leg cramp pain on walking)
- Arrhythmia (irregular heart beat)
- Diabetic retinopathy
- Macular degeneration of the eye
- Osteoarthritis
- Kidney stones
- Symptoms of senility
- Tinnitus (ringing in the ears) if due to reduced circulation.

Other benefits often reported:
- Reduction of diabetic complications
- Improved eyesight (small cataracts disappear)
- Increased warmth and strength
- Improved heart function
- Improved memory
- Parkinsons symptoms reduced
- Improved sense of well being

- Improved skin texture and tone
- Improved sexual function

Internet site: For further information you may care to visit an internet site: http://www.box.net.au/~rick. This site has links to a site that has answers to many other questions you may have.

ACNEM

The Australasian College of Nurtritional & Environmental Medicine (ACNEM) operates a free patient referral service, where people can be directed to doctors in Australia and New Zealand who have been trained in nutritional and environmental medicine by ACNEM. The service operates 10 am and 4 pm, Monday to Friday. Tel: (03) 9589 6088. Mail enquiries: 13 Hilton Street, Beaumaris VIC 3193. Fax: (03) 9589 5158. e-mail: acnem@mail.austasia.net. Information about ACNEM is available at their web site: http://www.acnem.org/.

Arcadia Health Centre

For supervised fasting, the Arcadia Health Centre caters for this. The following details outline the Centre.

ARCADIA HEALTH CENTRE PHILOSOPHY

Hygiene, as a system of health care, evolved and developed in the United States. It emphasises the fundamental importance of lifestyle management (bionomics) in the maintenance and recovery of health.

Hygiene, as a philosophy, teaches that healing is a biological process, the function of which is dependant upon the appropriate provision of the basic needs of life, that is, food, air, water, sunshine, rest, sleep, activity, mental and emotional influences etc.

In the practical care of the sick, Arcadia use only conservative means. No drugs or surgery are employed. Only those materials and influences which have a normal relationship to the organism are provided. Their first objective in attempting to restore normal physiological function is to remove, as far as practicable, the known causes of disease: faulty diet, inadequate activity, poison habits, physical and psychological stress, biomechanical factors and other aspects of lifestyle which influence physical and psychological well-being.

They believe it is largely ignorance which prevents us from realising that nearly all disease evolves from a combination of physical and psychological factors, many of which are within our own voluntary control.

There is no blue print programme which will satisfy everyone's needs. Each person requires care appropriate to their own requirements. Care cannot be effective if applied according to some arbitrary standard without recourse to individual capacity.

Emphasis on the hygienic approach is health orientated rather than disease orientated, that is, the focus is on health care and the removal of the causes of disease, rather than the vigorous and active treatment of disease which often involves the use of substances and procedures in themselves inimical to health.

FACILITY

The Centre is peacefully located in the beautiful Hills District 40 kilometres from Sydney, and provides an excellent environment for the effective application of conservative care.

Whether one needs close personal supervision for a chronic health problem, specialised care of back and joint pains, safe and effective weight reduction or merely the incentive to rest, recuperate and modify ones lifestyle, Arcadia's professional staff will assist in education, care and recovery.

The centre was designed and built for its current purposes. The rooms and amenities facilitate the application of hygienic care with natural light, fresh air, through ventilation, easy access and energy conserving utilities. Beauty and cleanliness are positive factors in the restoration and preservation of health.

The units are private or semi-private, each with adjoining facilities. The grounds are attractive and spacious with a swimming pool and spa. Bicycles and apparatus are available for other activities.

The total environment is intended to provide the most favourable conditions for rest, of vital importance to recuperation and recovery.

PROCEDURES

On admission, a complete case history is taken followed by a physical and biomechanical examination, Stress ECG, spirometry and other tests may be performed. All conventional X-ray, pathology services and darkfield microscopy are available.

Following the initial consultation and health assessment, a full disclosure is made and an open discussion ensues to determine the appropriate care and the means whereby the goals may be realised. The emphasis is on individual care.

The technique of fasting may be applied under close supervision, followed by a carefully planned nutritional programme to potentiate the body's immune system.

Health care is self care. Our educational programme ensures that each person learns how to care for themselves intelligently and responsibly to preserve and protect their health. On discharge an individualised outline of management is provided and where practicable follow-up consultations enable modifications to be introduced.

OUTPATIENTS

Out-patient facilities are conducted at the clinic and at The MLC Medical Centre (Corner, King and Castlereagh Street, Sydney). These are staffed by registered chiropractors and osteopaths and certified members of the International Association of Professional Hygienists. The service of a graduate psychologist is also available.

Consultations are by appointment only.

TRAINING

The Australian College of Hygiene Pty Ltd (non-profit) is a graduate training facility recognised by the International Association of Professional Hygienists Inc. Ohio, USA.

Suitable, licensed health professionals are required to undergo a minimum period of six months internship full-time to acquire certification by the Association.

The Arcadia Health Centre can be contacted on Tel: (02) 9653 1115 or (02) 9653 2678.

Ian Gawler

Dr Ian Gawler, one of Australia's best known cancer survivors and advocates of 'health and peace of mind' is a veterinarian and decathlete from Melbourne. In 1975 he developed cancer and lost a leg, but overcame the disease when it returned with effective self-help techniques that Ian and his wife developed.

Ian is also the therapeutic director of The Gawler Foundation — an organisation established in 1983 for people affected by cancer which has now blossomed into a dynamic life-force in health, healing and well-being.

The Foundation, based in Victoria's beautiful Yarra Valley, offers credential & ongoing programs to provide active support and self-help techniques for people affected by cancer, as well as programs which address disease-prevention, stress management, self-healing and the pursuit of meaning, purpose and truth. These programs attract people from all over Australia as well as overseas.

For further information contact Tel: (03) 59 671730.

Stephen Taylor

Stephen has been through the trauma of a brain tumour, worked as a counsellor at the Cancer Care Centre before being employed by Ian Gawler at Yarra Junction. He has had extensive experience with meditation, interpretation of drawings, counselling, group work etc.

Stephen now lives and works in Clare, South Australia with his wife Edeltraud Ennich and their two daughters.

8 day course (by donation):
Once a month, Sunday to Sunday for up to 12 people per course. Accommodation can be arranged nearby with healthy meals provided.

Weekend meditation retreat
($85 food & accommodation, plus donation):
Quarterly, Friday night to Sunday afternoon, at Sevenhill Retreat House. Contact re: dates.

Counselling (by donation): One to one available.

For further information contact Tel: (08) 8842 3114.

164

CHILDREN AND FOOD

Since my family and I have changed our diet the most often asked question, especially from mothers is, "What do you feed your children?".

It seems that if we take away meat, dairy and pasta, we are left with nothing to feed them. Of course, this is far from the truth. When Anna and I returned from Mexico, the first thing I did was empty out our pantry of all snack foods. Biscuits, chips, lollies, chocolate, crackers, fruit bars, canned foods, anything that contained preservatives and was processed. I also cleaned out our freezer of any frozen produce, including frozen vegetables and meat.

Also I would like to stress that when cleaning out our cupboards we asked our children to participate. It was very important for them to understand why we were doing this. They were quite happy to help. It doesn't mean that all of a sudden they get over their munchies because they don't. For several days later they would cry and whinge for a lolly or chips, but of course there were none to be found, so they would be satisfied with what there was in the house, in this case, fresh fruit and vegetables.

From when Olivia and Christian were very young their breakfast would consist mainly of milk and cereal. Snack time would be a fruit bar or a snack size pack of chips and a glass of lemonade. Lunch would consist of processed cheese and crackers, sometimes with a carrot thrown in for good measure, and of course more milk which they loved. Snack time again, lollies, chocolates, whatever their little hands could get a hold of. Dinner would alternate between meat and pasta.

It is very important that we offer our children alternatives in their diets. Also presentation of their food is very important. When giving them fruit and vegetables, especially if they have never really been keen on them, don't just give them a carrot or a whole apple. Prepare a platter for them. We generally slice up an apple into thin slices, together with carrot sticks, celery sticks, chopped up capsicum, strawberries and also dried fruits and nuts. Sure, it takes time, but it's sure worth it when you see your genetic immortality thriving.

Upon presentation of this platter children love seeing all the colour and you will soon discover that they will eat everything.

Taking away their milk was one of the hardest things to do because Christian especially, loved and lived on milk. But his love was also his downfall, because it contributed to his asthma and mucus congestion. We replaced the milk with soya milk. They did not immediately start drinking it by the glass full, so to help the transition along, we mixed a little soya milk with their milk until they finally acquired a taste for the soya. Instead of sweet biscuits they have porridge, Vita Brits, Rice Flakes or Bran Cereal bought in bulk from our health shop. They alternate mornings with wholemeal toast or a boiled egg. Before their breakfast they always have 1/2 teaspoon of vitamin C powder mixed with either orange, grape or apple juice. This has become a ritual for them and they no longer quibble when they are given their vitamins and juices. As I stated earlier on with Christian, he has had no asthma attacks since. If they seem to come down with a little sniffle, we immediately pump them up with fresh fruit and vegetable juices, Vitamin C and Echinacea which is available from health stores and is extremely good for flus and colds. As with all medication, Echinacea should not be taken for a prolonged period as it is taxing on the liver. This regime seems to stop the cold in its tracks. In times where they have had a little fever, instead of rushing for antibiotics as in the past, we keep their bodies cool with a damp flannel and monitor their temperature. Their immune system helps fight any infection which they may have had and their temperature returns to normal. It goes to prove that if you feed your body with the right foods, your immune system will be prepared to attack any foreign virus or bacteria it may encounter.

The children go to school, so in their lunch boxes they have a salad sandwich, one or two pieces of fruit, some nuts and dried fruits and a bottle of spring water. We no longer have any bottled drinks in the house. Snack times for the kids is always raw vegetables and fruit. As treats we sometimes let them have a packet of organic corn chips which are made without salt. For dinner we have a bowl of soup (minestrone style), baked potatoes, salad, steamed vegetables and some brown rice. Because the kids tend to graze all day, dinner is never a big deal. Basically, if we feel hungry, we eat. If we don't then we have a juice and a piece of fruit with a cup of herbal tea before bed. They have truly embraced their camomile and peppermint teas.

Some may think that what I have mentioned is a bit basic and how can they have this diet day in and day out. What I have come to learn over time is that children like variety in their diets and of course they love their treats. Unfortunately in many children's diets today, treats have become everyday foods. Although we abolished all snack foods from the house, the children still do enjoy them but they have come to appreciate them once again as treat foods. They mainly receive their treat foods when visiting their grandparents or when invited to birthday parties.

Gerson stated that by eating 75% healthy, then 25% was acceptable to splash out, if you wish. Meaning, if you eat at least five to six days of healthy, freshly prepared meals, then you can indulge in other foods, knowing that your body is healthy and able to digest them.

Together with Anna, we have listed below, a few recipes which are quick and simple to prepare for children and adults alike.

POTATO CHIPS

Wash and scrub desired amounts of potatoes required. Thinly slice potatoes and place them on an oven rack and bake till golden brown and crisp. Children love these and they feel that they are not missing out on their packet chips and they are a whole lot more nutritious for them.

POTATO WEDGES

Wash and scrub potatoes and cut into wedges. Place in non stick tray or dish and bake till golden brown. You can serve these with a yoghurt dip.

YOGHURT DIP

250ml plain yoghurt
250ml German style quark (available in organic or health stores)
2 diced spring onions
Crushed garlic

Blend yoghurt and quark together. Add spring onion and desired amount of crushed garlic. Very tasty and refreshing.

FISH

Olivia in particular seems to adjust her palate to any food presented to her, whereas Christian is a little more hesitant. The fish that we mostly eat is deep sea fish which are highly mineralised and do not contain pollutants that some fresh water fish contain. After rinsing it in clean spring water, with lemon juice, we either grill or poach the fish and serve it with freshly chopped parsley, pure olive oil and crushed garlic. Olivia loves it and Christian is just starting to have a couple of mouthfuls. As the saying goes "It won't happen overnight, but it WILL happen!".

Another way we prepare the fish, so as to add variety and get our little man of the house to eat it without realising that it is fish, is to cut it up into small bite sizes, baste them in a beaten egg, then crumb them and lightly bake them. Christian calls them 'Fishchickenees'.

SOUPS

Soups have never been a great favourite with our children except if it contains little noodles in a broth. They tend to cringe if they see big chunks of vegetables in there. So the best solution is to puree all your soups.

Pumpkin Soup
Pumpkin, Potatoes, Carrots, Celery, Onions, Leek

Peel and coarsely chop up onions and place them in a stainless steel or cast iron pot. (It retains all the flavours of the vegetables). Wash and chop all the other vegetables and pile on top, adding enough water to cover all the vegetables. Let the vegetables simmer very slowly for approximately 1 to 1.5 hours, keeping an eye on the water level and occasionally stirring. When tender, puree in the pot itself and switch off heat.

Amounts of vegetables will depend on the quantity of soup you desire, pumpkin and potatoes being the predominant vegetable.

Tomato Soup
Tomatoes, Leek, Onions

Celery

As with the above soup, wash, scrub and dice the vegetables and cover with enough water. With this soup in particular, do not add too much water, as the onions supply a lot of moisture and it is better to add extra water than to have too much.

Cabbage and celery

Cabbage, Celery, Onions, Leeks

As with the above soups, once again the preparation is the same. Puree at the completion of cooking. Salt is not added to any of our soups as celery is very high in natural sodium, therefore we use celery as a base for all our soups.

Of course there are so many different variations of vegetable soups, you need only use your imagination and remember, adding onions and celery, provide moisture and taste. Barley is also another very good base to add to soups.

OATMEAL COOKIES

75g unsalted butter, chopped
2 tablespoons honey
2 tablespoons boiling water
1 teaspoon low allergy baking powder
3/4 cup brown rice flour
3/4 cup rolled oats
3/4 cup dark brown raw sugar or honey
1/2 cup raisins or chopped up dried apricots
1/2 cup chopped carob bits.

1. Combine butter and honey in a small pan, stir over a low heat until butter is melted. Combine water and baking powder in a small glass and add to butter mixture; mix well, and let cool.

2. Sift flour into a bowl, add oats, sugar, raisins and carob bits; stir in butter mixture.

3. Roll level tablespoons of mixture into balls. Place balls about 8cm apart on greased oven trays. Lightly press balls to flatten slightly.

4. Cook in a slow oven, 150°C, for about 18 minutes or until browned. Stand cookies on trays for 2 minutes before placing on wire racks to cool. Store in an airtight container. Kids love them!

The above recipes are only a guideline. There are so many versatile dishes and so many good recipe books on the market catering for healthy eating and vegetarian dishes. Use organic produce as much as possible. Remember that most important of all when it comes to children it is the presentation, and the more raw vegetables and salads, the better!

FOOD

At the beginning of the therapy we were very strict and would only consume fruits and vegetables. Occasionally the kids would have some free range chicken. As I progressed, we started introducing other foods into our diet, specifically brown rice, legumes, pulses, fish, low fat yoghurt, quark, tofu and non-yeast breads. I suppose that as a Gerson patient, it was hard for me personally to sit and watch the others consume foods I had been raised on all my life, so to make it more enjoyable for me to consume my meals Anna and the kids would eat what I did, which made life a whole lot easier. You may think this a little unfair. But consider this. If your child were sick and needed to change his or her diet, I am quite certain that nearly every parent would eat the same food as their child. If undertaking the Gerson Therapy it is important to make the patient eat and enjoy their meals, for it is an essential part of their recovery. As with children, presentation of meals and variety is very important. Also sitting and enjoying their meal is the greatest medicine of all, because you are showing that you really love them and believe in what they are doing, and besides, you are totally rebuilding and helping your own body before an illness has a chance to attack it.

If you bite the bullet and take on the challenge of gaining control of your own body and nourishing it with the right foods, the end result will be nothing short of a miracle. The strict restriction of protein at the beginning was only for a short while, and we gradually introduced different foods. All the vital information is contained in "A Cancer Therapy". I was very strict with myself and never swayed. As time went on, I learnt to listen to my body and started adjusting my eating habits accordingly. We started experimenting with different ways to make oatmeal for breakfast. We varied the ways in which we prepared our soups and vegetables and we soon discovered that we preferred eating our vegetables raw most of the time. Eventually fish came into the diet and we now have fish twice a week. Green salads are also a base of our everyday meals. Anna and the kids still indulge in other food on weekends. The basis to our eating habits is once again 75% healthy, 25% social eating.

The diet we currently follow is contained within Ian Gawler's book, "You Can Conquer Cancer" and also Kathryn Alexander's book "Get A Life" *(See Book Review, pages 225, 229)*. Both these books contain excellent dietary information.

We have been asked umpteen times by friends and family members, how can you possibly eat this bland food, day in day out? I suppose you could call it bland when you first start out but soon it becomes very enjoyable and whenever you do indulge in 'tasty food' you will soon discover the way your body reacts. At times when Anna has indulged, she has said to me that her taste buds went wild, but later her digestion suffered the consequences. There are so many good health cook books on the market, but one in particular I would like to mention, is called 'Recipes For Longer Life' by Ann Wigmore, (© 1978 by Ann Wigmore and Hippocrates Health Institute, Avery Publishing Group Inc, Wayne, New Jersey USA). The following statement which I feel sums up the connection between life and nutrition as quoted in her book is:

"Recipes for Life is for Every man and Every woman and Every child who feels that there can be more to life than presently experienced. The RECIPES FOR LIFE people say, "Eat as if your life depended on it ... it does!". Eat "God's greatest hits" ... whole foods, live foods, healthy foods, life-giving food ... and then witness the incredible health benefits that these foods bestow upon us all!"

You will find a multitude of quick and easy recipes to not only feed, but nourish your family. The book covers recipes from entrees to desserts, including dips and juices using all 'live food ingredients'. Ann Wigmore has over 15 books in publication.

A few easy meal preparations which we use are listed as follows:

OATMEAL

Rolled oats or oatmeal with dried apricots, prunes and raisins

Before going to bed, place approx. 7 apricots and 4 prunes and a handful of raisins into a pot and cover with water. In another pot, place one cup of oats and cover with water. Upon rising the next day, cook fruits for approximately 10 minutes, at the same time cooking the oats. Combine oats and fruits together and enjoy! Makes enough for two. You may want to use a little honey. Vary fruits to your preference, eg. pears, peaches etc.

Alternate oatmeal with fresh fruit salad mixed with soya yoghurt.

SALAD

When it comes to salads, everything goes. The more vegetables, the more substance a salad has. We use a combination of:

Cos lettuce, Butter lettuce, Endive, Fennel, Carrot, Alfalfa sprouts, Broccoli, Cauliflower, Cabbage, Mung beans, Chickpeas

Wash and drain all the lettuce leaves. Shred the carrot and cabbage into a bowl. Finely chop the fennel, broccoli, cauliflower and add into the bowl. Tear the lettuce leaves into small pieces and add to bowl. Sprinkle alfalfa over the top. Squeeze one or two lemons into salad with approximately 1 tablespoon of flax seed oil. The taste is truly unique. Of course salads vary depending on availability of vegetables. Alternatives for dressing are apple cider vinegar or red wine vinegar and a little olive oil. These are very simple dressing ideas which we prefer to all others and they are not as heavy as some.

OUR SPECIAL VINAIGRETTE

3 tblspns apple cider vinegar
1 tblspn flax seed oil
5 tblespns water
1 clove garlic and equal amount ginger crushed together
1 tspn honey

Mix ingredients together and pour over salad or great used as a dip with steamed vegetables.

YOHO DIP

We called this Yoho Dip because it is simply a mixture of non-fat yoghurt and homous. In a bowl place 3-4 tablespoons of yoghurt, add 1 tablespoon of homous and one of flax seed oil. You can add more or less homous according to your taste and according to quantity of dip required. Also a little crushed garlic and ginger is very good but of course optional. This dip makes a great topping for steamed vegetables or just served with pieces of toast or sticks of raw vegetables.

VIOLET DELIGHT

1 raw beetroot washed and peeled
1 carrot washed and peeled
2 tablespoons yoghurt
1 teaspoon flax seed oil

Finely grate carrot and beetroot into a bowl. Add yoghurt and flax seed oil. Enjoy!

HIPPOCRATES SOUP

This is the main important dish in the Gerson diet. Hippocrates was a Greek physician who lived some four hundred years before the birth of Christ. He was the Father of Medicine who taught that live food could restore and maintain vibrant health. He affirmed that "your food shall be your medicine, and your medicine shall be your food."

2 potatoes, scrub and cut into quarters with skin
2 sticks of celery diced
1 leek diced
2 tomatoes cut
small bunch of parsley chopped.

Boil one litre of spring water in a stainless steel or cast iron pot, then add vegetables and simmer on low heat for approximately 1.5-2 hours. Put through a food mill adding a little water until achieving the consistency of thickness you require.

OUR SOUP

2 onions
3 medium carrots
3 sticks celery
1 sweet potato
3 cloves garlic
3 potatoes
string beans (desired amounts: approx. 2 handfuls)
1 small red or green capsicum

Peel and dice all vegetables into a large heavy pot (cast iron preferable). Slice garlic into pot. Pour in 3 glasses of spring water (approx. 900ml). Cover soup and put on low heat for approx. 2 hours, stirring occasionally. Serve with a sprinkle of cayenne pepper and a dash of pure olive oil.

SWEET POTATOES

Wash and scrub 4 sweet potatoes, then make small cuts with a knife and place in a baking dish. Pour 1/2 glass of freshly squeezed orange juice over the top and 1 tablespoon of honey for taste. Cover and place in a 180°C oven and cook for approximately one hour. Check from time to time to ensure that there is enough moisture in the pan and turn potatoes for even cooking. The potatoes should be soft through the middle.

BANANA CAKE

4 cups of oatmeal
4 tablespoons of honey (to taste)
1/2 cup raisins
1/2 cup apple sauce (Granny Smith apples)
3 mashed bananas

Apple sauce: Peel and core 3 apples, slice and place in pan half-filled with water. Cook for approximately 15 minutes. Puree.

Mix all above ingredients together and pour into baking pan. Place in a pre-heated over at 250°C to start, then lower to 180°C to cook. Use fork or toothpick to check when it is cooked (approximately 45 mins). The centre shouldn't be wet. Great served with yoghurt or banana ice-cream.

BANANA ICE-CREAM

One of the most simple recipes would have to be banana ice-cream. Peel and freeze the required amount of bananas ensuring that they are ripe. Freeze for 24 hours. Once frozen put them through a Champion juicer with the blank plate in. The bananas will come out exactly like soft serve ice-cream. Kids and adults love it and you can combine it with other fruits like mango or strawberries. If you don't have a Champion juicer, you can put them through a blender.

The Champion Juicer is made in America and its operation is unique in the sense that it operates on the mastication process. The Champion chews the fibres and breaks up the cells of vegetables and fruits, which produces more live enzymes, vitamins and trace minerals. The results are a, richer colour, sweeter and more full-bodied juice.

It has been used successfully for over 30 years to assist people undergoing the Gerson and other nutritional based therapies.

The Champion is a very simple juicer to use. With just a few changes, it becomes three machines in one. As well as extracting juices, the unit can make coconut milk, baby foods, fruit sauces, nut butters, grated vegetables and nuts, and of course ice-cream.

The Champion Juicer is not available in retail stores. If you would like more information and prices, write or fax to:

Living Proof
PO Box 377, Magill SA 5072. Tel: (08) 8364 4925
The above recipes are only a few simple ones. There are so many and the good thing is that even the Gerson patient can enjoy them!

You will notice that most of the recipes above, all contain Flax Seed Oil. Since we use it everyday, I would like to elaborate on it a little more.

WHAT IS FLAX SEED OIL

Flax oil is our richest source of the valuable omega-3, -6 & -9 fatty acids. Flax oil contains 50%-60% of the Omega-3 which is almost twice as much as those found in fish oils, which go up to around 30% maximum. Research and clinical experience have shown beneficial effects in so many areas such as:

Heart Disease: Omega-3's lower high blood cholesterol and triglyceride levels by as much as 25% and 65% respectively. Max Gerson used flax oil for its cholesterol-lowering effect.

Cancers: Omega-3's dissolve tumours. Max Gerson also used the flax oil for this purpose. Dr Budwig in Germany has over 1,000 documented cases of successful cancer treatment using flax oil along with additional nutritional support. She has been using it successfully in cancer therapy for over 30 years.

Asthma: Flax oil can relieve asthma noticeably, sometimes within a few days of starting the oil.

Water retention: Flax oil helps the kidney remove sodium and water. Water retention (oedema) is involved in swollen ankles, some forms of obesity, PMS, and late stages of cancer and cardiovascular disease.

There are so many areas in which flax oil is also beneficial. To know more about the Flax oil, go to your local health shop where they keep it in stock and also pick up a nutritional guide pamphlet by Udo Erasmus, Author of "Fats and Oils" and "Fats that Heal, Fats that Kill", or you can write to Stoney Creek Oil Products Pty Ltd, Talbot VIC 3371. Tel: (054) 63 2340.

DAIRY

Many of you may want to know a little more about the milks available. Dairy products were temporarily removed from Christians diet for approximately 12 months as they were the most significant cause of Christian's congestion and asthma. We occasionally have goat and sheep cheese. These cheeses do have a stronger taste to them, but to our amazement Christian took a liking to them. Goat's milk contains more calcium, iron, proteins and vitamins than cow's milk. It is more digestible by the human body. Cow's milk is for babies only, as the enzymes required to digest it disappear from the human body at 3 years of age. Goat's milk is an ideal health food as it is allergy free and it is the closest to human milk and is suitable for babies. It is available as cheese, yoghurt and also ice-cream and is available in most organic and health stores.

Vegetable nutritional guide

To overcome the effects of stress, pollution and fast food we require far more vitamins, minerals and living enzymes than the recommended daily allowance currently suggests.

The best way to obtain these vitamins, minerals and enzymes in large amounts is to simply drink fresh juice. And the best juice to drink should be extracted by a juicer that removes fibre (which requires digestion) so that all the nutrients are absorbed straight into the bloodstream for immediate effect.

While on the intense Gerson Therapy, we used the Norwalk Juicer (purchased in the United States). This machine is the ultimate in juicers, as it grinds and presses separately, giving a smooth and rich juice. To date we have not found a distributor within Australia but should you be interested in purchasing a Norwalk Juicer, we have included an order form on *page 116*. As mentioned, the Champion Juicer is much easier to use, and is readily available, however, it does not produce the amount or quality of juice to that of the Norwalk Juicer. When we purchased the Norwalk juicer, we received a book to illustrate its use and also the contents in various vegetables and fruits when juicing.

I would therefore like to pass on the following information to you as extracted from the Norwalk Juicer manual:

From official publications of the United States Department of Agriculture we have compiled tables of vitamin and mineral content which you will find for most of the commodities.

We emphasise that the nutrient values given are only representative of a great number of individual samples which have been analysed. The values contained in any particular food which you might buy for your table could vary widely depending on such factors as variety, breed, soil factors, seasonal and geographic differences, state of maturity, length of time since harvested and method of storage.

AFALFA

Named 'Al-Fal-Fa' meaning Father of All Foods. One of the oldest cultivated plants, it has been used for thousands of years for forage and grazing.

Its roots can go down 40 feet or more to extract minerals usually available only to trees. Has the highest nutrient content of any plants used for livestock. It is rich in Vitamins A, B1, B6, B12, C, D, E, K, biotin, folic acid, niacin and pantothenic acid. Also minerals (copper, iron, magnesium, phosphorous, calcium-twice the content of powdered whole milk-potassium, magnesium, iron and enzymes critical for food assimilation).

It is the highest of all leafy vegetables in protein with 20% of the dried plant composed of digestible protein as compared with 27% in whole milk powder.

It is an excellent source of fibre, up to 50% by weight compared with less than 10% in wheat bran. It contains saponims, sterols, flavinoids, coumarins, alkaloids and acids. It is one of the richest foods we have in chlorophyll.

Overall it is one of the most nutritious foods known. In the British Herbal Pharmacopoeia, alfalfa is recognised as a convalescent remedy for debility and also as a therapeutic treatment for deficiencies of Vitamins A, C, E and K.

Alfalfa is repeatedly referred to in its literature as being a 'tonic'. It is called a kidney tonic, liver tonic, restorative tonic, digestive tonic, prostate tonic, reproductive tonic, muscle tonic and gland tonic, among others. Alfalfa has been used in the treatment of many debilitating or degenerative diseases. It has a reputation as an appetite stimulant and vitality augmenter.

Some people might have toxic reactions to large quantities of alfalfa juice. For this reason we suggest that it be taken in small quantities mixed with other juices. Health food stores carry alfalfa in powder, tablet and other forms as a food supplement and as a tea made from the leaves and seeds of the plant.

ALMONDS (Prunus amygdalus)

Many vegetarians make almonds an important part of their diet because gram for gram they contain more protein than sirloin steak. They also contain much more fat. But the fat is mostly unsaturated with a good amount of lineoleic acid which helps lower blood pressure and is a factor in maintaining a healthy cardiovascular system. They also carry a good supply of B vitamins, vitamin E, magnesium, iron and fibre.

APPLES (Malus sylvestris)

Some are an important source of Vitamin C. Also B1, B2, B6, niacin, carotene, biotin and folic acid. Also high in pectin, malic acid and tannic acid for purifying the intestinal area. Apple juice is a blood purifier, a general tonic and is helpful to the skin. It is good for flushing the kidneys and controlling digestive upsets.

APRICOTS (Prunis armenaica)

A favourite food of the Hunzas, people renowned for their longevity who live in the Himalayan mountains. They are used on space flights as puddings and as part of snack bars for energy and high nutrient content.

Apricots contain Vitamins A, B, C, beta carotene (an excellent source), protein, lipids, trace elements including magnesium, phosphorous, iron, calcium, potassium, sodium, sulphur, manganese, cobalt and bromine. If you crack the apricot pit open and eat the nut inside you will have an important addition of nitrilosides and Vitamin B17 (laetrile).

ASPARAGUS (Asparagus officinalus)

Look for firm, straight stalks with well formed, tightly closed tips. Try to use within 2-3 days.

Asparagus contains rutin, a bioflavinoid which contributes to the health of the small capillaries. Also aspargine, an alkaloid which in raw juice stimulates the kidneys causing a strong diuretic effect as well as a strong odour and colour to the urine which is not a matter for concern. Only a small amount of the juice need be taken for this effect. The green varieties contain much more nutrient than the white.

Asparagus contains a good amount of Vitamin C, A, and B-Complex. Also potassium, manganese and iron.

AVOCADO (Persea species)

Originally from Mexico and Central America. It is very high in protein, much more like a nut than a fruit. It contains a large supply of beta carotene (3 times as much ripe as unripe), 11 vitamins and 17 minerals for a high level of nutrition. Third highest amount of fruits in oil content, free of cholesterol and easy to assimilate. The avocado is high in Vitamins A, D and E.

For immediate use select slightly soft avocados, free of blemishes and dark spots. For later use get hard to firm ones which should ripen at home at room temperature in a few days. When ripe they may be refrigerated, but plan to use them within three to five days. Store at room temperature in paper bags if you wish to speed up ripening.

Avocado oil is an excellent penetrating oil when used as an emollient, ideal for soothing sensitive skin.

BANANAS (Musa paradisiaca)

Bananas contain practically no fat, have a moderate calorie count and are extremely low in sodium. They are rich in essential vitamins and minerals, high in potassium and a good source of Vitamin B6, magnesium and manganese. Bananas help maintain nourishment and weight. They are used in pregnancies, 1 or 2 bananas daily promote better retention of nitrogen, phosphorous, calcium and other elements important for building new tissues.

A good solid food for infants and aged. They are helpful in correcting protein deficiencies. Paediatricians often spoon feed as a first solid food for babies, and also to help with their gastro-intestinal disorders. Used in cases of celiac disease in infants. Helps digestive upsets in the aged. It's an anti-diarrhoel agent, useful in illness. It builds iron stores and is soothing for kidneys and peptic ulcers.

Banana pectin swells causing voluminous soft bland cleanout of intestines along with bacteria absorbed by the pectin.

When bananas are green tipped, use them for cooking; when all yellow, for cooking or eating. When they are flecked with brown spots they are fully ripe, perfect for infant feeding, ideal for blending into cakes, cookies, breads, puddings, and milk shakes.

BEANS (Phaseolus)

Contain Vitamins A, B-Complex, C, Inositol, chlorophyll and minerals including phosphorus, calcium, copper and cobalt. Said to promote normal action of liver and pancreas. Used by some in quantities of 4oz per day or so of the juice for rheumatism, gout and as a diuretic.

BEETROOTS (Beta vulgaris)

Amino acids are present in good quantity. Also salts of phosphorous, sodium, calcium, potassium and magnesium. A combination of beetroot and carrot juice furnishes a good percentage combination of the above plus sulphur as well as a high concentration of Vitamin A.

An excellent diuretic, toner and builder. Beetroot juice should be started with small amounts, gradually building up to larger quantities. Please note: Starting with larger amounts could cause dizziness or nausea.

BEETROOT LEAVES

As others of the leafy greens, contains a large amount of beta carotene, more potassium by weight than bananas. A good source of Vitamin C, iron and magnesium.

BLUEBERRIES (Vaccinium species)

They are now second only to strawberries as being our most popular berry. Next to wheat bran they are the highest source of manganese in one study of 120 other foods. They are also a good source of Vitamin A, potassium and other of the micro nutrients.

BRAZIL NUTS (Bertholletia excelsa)

Brazil nuts are very high in fat. They also contain good amounts of calcium, phosphorous, iron, potassium, magnesium and the B vitamins.

BROCCOLI (Brassica oleraca var. botrytis)

Look for broccoli stalks that are tender and firm with tightly closed flower buds. They will keep for three to five days in the crisper or put in plastic bags. This member of the cabbage family is at the top of the list for vitamin and mineral concentration. It is very low in calories and sodium.

BRUSSEL SPROUTS

Brussel sprouts should be small, firm and compact. If they smell strong they are probably too old.

Member of the brassica (cabbage) family. One of the top sources of Vitamin C containing gram for gram, 1/3 more than oranges. High in Vitamin A, some of the B-Complex and potassium. Many nutritionists believe that a combination of the juice of brussel sprouts, string beans, lettuce and carrot furnishes elements needed to strengthen and regenerate certain functions of the pancreas.

BUCKWHEAT (Fagopyrum esculentum)

Buckwheat is grain like, but not a grain. Unlike wheat, rice and other grains it has no bran or germ, but consists only of a shell with a kernel inside. The kernel is called a 'groat'. It is the edible part of the buckwheat.

Buckwheat has the best protein quality of any of the grain. It is high in the amino acid lycine where other grains are low. Combining with other grains creates a very high quality protein. It is also rich in B6 containing 40% more than whole wheat, 76% more than dry oatmeal, 57% more than cornmeal and 60% more than barley. Also a good source of other B vitamins providing more thiamine and riboflavin than whole wheat. It has more than twice the iron contained in brown rice and is a fairly good source of potassium. Because few insects attack it, it is usually grown without insecticides.

It is the best vegetable source of protein (between 11-15%) having about the same nutrient efficiency as proteins of animal origin with a high biological value. It is high in manganese which is essential for muscle control, healthy growth and reproductive systems, good metabolism and the activation of enzymes.

Buckwheat is the best know source of rutin. It is extraordinarily rich in magnesium which is vital for the utilisation of many vitamins.

CABBAGE (Brassica oleracea var. capitala)

A member of the brassica family. Loaded with vitamins and other nutrients. Combats nutritional deficiencies, boosts energy, improves chemical reactions within the body. One of the most beneficial foods known to man. The raw juice is used extensively by ulcer patients.

It is high in sulphur, calcium, phosphorous, iodine, magnesium, potassium, iron and copper. Also in Vitamin A, B1, B2 and chlorophyll.

Much of the nutrient in cabbage is lost in cooking, so it is best to eat it raw or in the form of raw juice.

CARROTS (Daucus carota var. sativa)

Extremely high in beta carotene which is a precursor to Vitamin A. Beta carotene is stored in the liver and is converted to Vitamin A as needed by the body. Diabetics sometimes have trouble making the conversion and might have to get their Vitamin A from fish liver oils.

Carrot juice provides energy, is a good source of minerals, helps promote normal elimination, aids diuresis, helps build healthy tissue, skin and teeth. It helps prevent eye infections, contributes to the general health of the optic system, helps treatment of ulcers and furnishes vital enzymes to body tissues.

Try to get the freshest, largest and most mature carrots possible. According to government reports the Vitamin A values of the principal varieties of carrots will run from 7,000 to 12,000 international units per hundred grams are usually harvested for use as fresh vegetables. These values will increase to 17,000 to 38,000 international units at the maximum state of maturity deemed acceptable. In other words, the larger the carrots, the higher the per gram content of both juice and nutrients.

In order to make it possible to store carrot juice for several days it is necessary to peel the carrots in order to remove the soil bacteria which cause spoilage.

While many people believe that a large part of the nutrient content of the potato is contained in or just under the skin, most people are surprised to find that this is not true with the carrot. With the carrot there is little, if any, more nutrient in or under the skin than in the rest of the carrot. The carrot should be cut off just under the green dirt ring at the top and the tail removed.

CASHEWS (Anacardium occidentale)

The cashew instead of being a nut is actually the seed of a fruit called the cashew apple.

There is no such thing on the market as 'raw' cashews. All cashews for human consumption have to be heated to expel naturally occurring toxins. If you enjoy the flavour of roasted cashews, you lose little nutritive value by roasting them lightly in your oven. Cashews are high in phosphorous, iron, potassium, magnesium and the B vitamins.

CAULIFLOWER (Brassica oleracea var. botrytis)

Because of its low content it is a favourite of dieters. Its abundance of fibre not only satisfies your hunger but promotes the health of your intestinal tract. Recent research indicates that cauliflower helps clear chemical pollutants from the body by activating certain enzyme systems.

CELERY (Apium graveolens)

Historically used by the ancients as a diuretic and laxative, to heal wounds, to soothe irritated nerves and to break up gallstones. Today it is used for problems of chemical imbalance and arthritis.

Celery has important concentrations of plant hormones and essential oils which give celery its strong characteristic smell. The oils have an effect on the regulation of the nervous system seeming to provide a calming effect.

Celery has also been used for its stimulating effect upon the sexual system. It is said to be particularly useful for a weak sex drive without increasing a normal drive.

A relaxing tonic at bedtime. Many drink it to help keep comfortable in hot weather.

Contains, Vitamins A, B-Complex, and C. Also a lot of sodium and good amounts of magnesium, manganese, iron, copper, potassium, calcium and phosphorous.

CHERRIES (Prunus species)

The dark cherries are said to have a higher nutritional value than the light ones because they have a higher content of iron, magnesium and silicon. They are valued as blood cleansers, as diuretics and for increasing the flow of digestive juices. They are effective cleansers of the liver and kidneys. In addition they have been used to alleviate discomfort of gout and arthritis.

CORN (Zea mays)

Corn is highly nutritious, easy to plant, quick to grow and can be readily stored for long periods of time.

DANDELION GREENS (Taraxicum officinale)

Dandelion contains 35% more Vitamin C than tomatoes and 20% more Vitamin A than carrots. It provides more calcium than soybeans, more iron than eggs, as much iron and twice as much thiamine as spinach, more potassium than kale and over 4 times as much riboflavin as lettuce. It is also rich in folic acid,

B-Complex, magnesium, calcium, sodium, silica and chlorophyll. Large, mature greens are better.

ENDIVE (Cichorium endiva)

Also known as escarole and chicory. It has elements needed by the optic system. 1 litre a day of a combination of endive, carrot, celery and parsley is said by some to help improve vision.

One of the richest sources of Vitamin A among green vegetables. Has been used in cases of hay fever and asthma as well as for liver and gall bladder dysfunction.

FENNEL (Foeniculum vulgare)

There are two kinds of fennel. One is the common or sweet fennel which is mainly used for condiments and flavouring. This is classified as a herb and is not recommended for use in juice form.

The second form is Florence Fennel, usually known as Finocchio which is used widely by Italians and other Latin peoples. This plant belongs to the celery family but its juice is much sweeter and more aromatic than celery juice. It contains an essential oil that soothes an irritated stomach. It helps in digestion and reduces flatulence.

Its juice is often combined with carrot juice as a tonic for the eyes. When beetroot juice is added it makes an excellent blood builder, helpful for anaemia caused by excessive menses. Use in moderation.

GRAPEFRUIT (Citrus paradisi)

Good appetiser, aids digestion, promotes diuresis, helps remove impurities from blood. Contains citric acid, sugars, pectins, essential oils including limonene, pimene and citrol, plus Vitamins C, A and P, plus calcium and phosphorous.

JERUSALEM ARTICHOKES (Helianthus tuberosus)

The tuber of a species of sunflower extensively grown in Italy and known there as the Archicioffo-Girasole (Girasole meaning Sunflower). Girasole was corrupted to Jerusalem when translated into English.

Because of a unique combination of enzymes this is said to be a tuber which diabetics can eat with impunity. Its juice is beneficial and palatable either alone or with other vegetables.

LEMONS (Citrus limon)

The lemon is at least 3,000 years old with its earliest known habitat being in Southeast Asia. Columbus carried lemon seeds on his second trip to the New World.

Whole books have been written about the multitude of different uses for lemons. When used as food they are a rich source of Vitamin C, bioflavinoids and Vitamin P, A and folic acid. Potassium, iron, magnesium and trace elements are also present along with a very low content of sodium.

LETTUCE

Vitamins: Beta carotene, C, D, E and B-Complex.

Minerals: Magnesium, calcium, Iodine, phosphorous, copper, cobalt, zinc and potassium.

Alkaloids: Asparagene lactucine, lactucuc acid and byoscyamine.

A large chlorophyll content is mostly in the outer green leaves.

ONIONS (Allium cepa)

Research studies have shown that both onion and garlic have the ability to reduce blood levels of cholesterol and triglycerides. People who eat significant quantities of them have healthier levels of blood fats than those who eat just a little. These foods also have a real ability to dissolve and prevent the type of blood clots associated with heart attacks and stroke.

If the taste of these foods are too strong for your comfort you many find that cooking reduces their strength to an acceptable level. Fortunately cooking does not seem to rob these foods of their cholesterol fighting potency.

ORANGES (Citrus sinensis)

Researchers say that orange juice protects you against colds and sore gums even better than ordinary Vitamin C. Doctors recommend it to patients with high blood pressure because of its plentiful content of potassium.

The orange is one of the world's most popular fruits. It probably originated in China and SE Asia. It then appeared in North Africa and Spain. Columbus took it to Haiti in 1493. Spanish and Portuguese explorers carried it to Florida and South America.

All oranges are tree ripened and many are ripe when they are green. They will not ripen after being picked. A temperature drop can cause an orange coloured orange to turn green.

Some growers will treat green oranges with ethiglene to decompose the chlorophyll and cause oranges to turn orange. Others also add dye and wax. Beware of perfect looking oranges. If they have green spots they are probably more natural.

In addition to the nutrients listed below, oranges also contain bioflavinoids, magnesium, copper, zinc, manganese and bromine.

PAPAYA (Carica papaya)

Papaya is full of proteolytic enzymes, the chemicals that make digestion easy. The principal one is papain which is commercially extracted and dried into powder for use as a digestant. It is also used as a meat tenderiser to help break down meat fibre. Papaya juice can be used by people with poor digestive ability. Older people in particular often used papaya to enhance digestion and assimilation.

Unripe papaya contains more digestive enzymes than ripe papaya. Papaya contains fiberin which is usually found only in animals and in man where it is part of the blood clotting mechanism. It also contains agrinine, thought to be good for male fertility, and carpain, thought to be good for the heart.

A wonderfully therapeutic drink can be made by combining papaya with pineapple juice which contains another digestive enzyme called bromelain. Papaya juice can also be combined with apple, pear or other fruit juices.

PARSLEY (Petroselinum crispum)

In ancient herbal practice parsley was used to build up strength, help sore eyes and bleeding gums. Parsley is one of the best sources of Vitamin A and high in Vitamin C, B-Complex and iron. It is also an excellent source of minerals.

Parsley affects oxygen metabolism, the urinary tract, capillary system, the eyes and optic nerve system (particularly when mixed with other juices) and the adrenal and thyroid glands. It is often given, along with dietary restrictions, to relieve menstrual problems. As a deodorant, parsley minimises the smell of onions, tobacco, liquor, etc. on the breath if taken at the same time. Parsley is easily grown indoors in a pot.

Select fresh green bunches without wilted or yellow leaves. Because of the structure of the plant it should be juiced or finely ground so that the many nutrients can be assimilated.

Parsley is a herb. The juice is very strong and rarely should be taken alone. In addition to the nutrients listed below, parsley contains oestrogens, chlorophyll, enzymes and minerals such as magnesium, sulphur, potassium, iodine, copper and manganese. Also essential oils: pinene, terpene, apial and apein.

PARSNIPS (Pastinaca saliva)

Used as a diuretic, an anti-arthritic and detoxifying agent.

The juice is low in calcium but rich in potassium, phosphorous, sulphur, silicon and chlorine. Do not confuse the organic chlorine which is important to the body with the chlorine used for disinfectant. Parsnip contains the rare combination of sulphur and silicon which is helpful to the strength and growth of nails and hair. It is particularly valuable in cases of brittle nails, and has also been helpful to an assortment of lung problems for which the unique combination of chlorine and phosphorous is helpful.

The parsnip should be cut off just under the dirt ring at the top and the tail should be removed. It should also be peeled.

PEACHES (Prunus persica)

Although originally from China this delicious fruit is now grown in temperate climates world wide. Low in calories for the diet conscious but high in flavour and Vitamin A.

PEAS (pisum sativum)

Snap peas are delicious when eaten or juiced raw, pods and all. They are rich in Vitamins A, C, niacin and some of the other B vitamins as well as minerals and fibre.

PEARS (Pyrus communis)

They are usually picked while green and should be set out for a few days to ripen slowly in a cool place. When ripened this way they are said to be less grainy. For quicker ripening they may be put in a closed paper bag. They should not be refrigerated until after they have ripened.

CAPSICUM PEPPERS GREEN, SWEET GARDEN VARIETIES (Capsicum annum)

Look for firm skins with bright colour (not pale or soft with thin skins). Wash, store in crisper or plastic bags. Use within a week.

The ingredient that makes members of the capsicum family hot is capsacin. Researchers believe that this also works to keep the blood from clotting which should be beneficial in cases of heart disorders.

The green pepper has a high content of Vitamin A and magnesium. In addition it contains more than twice as much Vitamin C as oranges.

PERSIMMONS (Diospyros virginiana)

High in Vitamin A and potassium. Select large, soft, well ripened fruit.

PINEAPPLE (Ananas pinea)

Buy good coloured pineapples. They do not ripen after being harvested. Watch for soft spots or brown leaves.

Pineapple contains a protein digestant called bromelain which is comparable in potency to pepsin and papain and can digest 1000 times its weight in protein.

The juice helps relieve discomfort of a sore throat and bronchitis and helps dissolve mucus formation. It also aids kidney function. In addition to the nutrients below, pineapple contains iodine, magnesium and sulphur. Also citric acid and malic acid.

Canned juices, even with no added sugar, loose 2/3 of their nutrient values.

POTATOES (Solanum tuberosum)

Potato juice is very soothing to the stomach and useful in cases of ulcers and gastritis — very cleansing — has been used in cases of gout. In addition to the nutrients given below potatoes also contain Vitamin K, folic acid, pantothenic acid, magnesium, manganese, copper and sulphur.

Procure well matured potatoes if possible. Wash well to remove all soil bacteria. If you peel them be sure to peel very lightly as a high concentration of vitamins and minerals is found directly under the skin. Beware of green potatoes, they are dangerous.

RADISHES (Raphanus sativus)

Radishes are very good for the body. They have a high alkali content which benefits the kidneys and bladder. They also supply a good quantity of sulfur and phosphorous. Black radishes contain Vitamin B1, C and E, magnesium and iodine plus large amounts of potassium and sodium. Pink radishes contain B-Complex, C, D, and P plus a sulfur compound, magnesium and iodine and also large amounts of potassium and sodium. The juice is too strong to take alone. It can be mixed with carrot juice to restore the tone of the mucous membranes. For a tonic effect you might try mixing and juicing 3 radishes and 1/2 onion with pineapple juice.

RASPBERRIES (Rubus species)

The raspberry has been used by man for at least 5,000 years both for delicious food and as a medicinal herb where the leaves and roots are used.

The fruit is rich in Vitamins A, C and B-Complex. It is also rich in tannin which is a natural astringent. Raspberries and their juice are used to tighten gums and mucous membranes being helpful in cases of gingivitis, diarrhoea and upset stomachs. The juice has long been used as a dentrifrice for the removal of plaque and tightening of gums

RHUBARB (Rheum rhaponticum)

Rhubarb has an extremely high content of oxalic acid. When cooked this acid is converted into an inorganic chemical which, when eaten, might deposit large amounts of oxalic acid crystals in the kidneys and other tissues. For this reason we do not recommend the used of cooked rhubarb.

Because of its supposed laxative qualities raw rhubarb juice in small quantities might have a beneficial effect.

RICE (Oryza sativa)

Rice feeds more than half of the world's people. All rice is originally brown. White rice is what is left when the bran is removed. The bran contains by far most of the minerals and the B vitamins thiamine, riboflavin, niacin. There is also a very large loss of chlorine, biotin, PABA and pyridoxine (vitamin B6). Brown rice is richer than wheat in protein, similar in B vitamins and has more iron, calcium and phosphorous. It is very high in potassium and low in sodium which makes it a favourite in cases of high blood pressure. It is easily digested and non-allergenic.

It has no Vitamin A or C. It has a high protein quality when combined with beans, legumes, seeds, nuts, etc.

SESAME SEED (Sesamum indicum)

Usually used to make tahini, a very nutritious seed butter. It is high in protein with large amounts of calcium, phosphorous, potassium and the B vitamins. It also provides an anti-oxidant, sesamol, which is believed by some researchers to slow aging and to help against cancer.

Store seeds in a cool dry place or refrigerate for longer storage.

SPINACH (Spinacia oleracea)

Raw spinach has long been regarded as one of the very finest agents for the cleansing, reconstruction and regeneration of the intestinal tract. For this reason, raw spinach and particularly raw spinach juice, is widely used for this purpose.

But when spinach is cooked or canned the oxalic acid content may be deposited in the kidneys and others tissues as oxalic acid crystals.

In addition to the nutrients listed below, spinach contains folic acid, oxalic acid, magnesium, sulfur, manganese, zinc, copper, iodine, chlorophyll and mucilage.

TANGERINES / MANDARIN ORANGES (Citrus reticulata)

Called Tangerines because these orange-like fruits were originally shipped to America from Tangiers in the early 1800s. They are sweeter than oranges and contain twice as much Vitamin A and considerably more Vitamin C. The mineral content is similar to the orange, the B vitamin content is lower.

TOMATOES (Lycopersicon esculentum)

The tomato is neither a vegetable nor a fruit. It is a berry. But by legal definition and common usage it is considered to be a vegetable and a popular one at that because they say it adds more nutrients to the diet than any other vegetable. But this is only because so many people like them as they only rank 16th in common vegetables in concentration of ten important vitamins and minerals.

TURNIP LEAVES (Brassica rapa)

Turnip leaves contain 90% of the nutrition in the turnip. They also contain a higher percentage of calcium than any other vegetable, an excellent source of organic calcium. Extremely high in Vitamins A, B, C and minerals. The root can be delicious sauteed in oil or in a stew. Some like it raw in salads.

In addition to the nutrients below, turnips contain sulfur, iodine and copper.

WALNUTS: ENGLISH AND BLACK (Juglans regia, juglans nigra)

Among the common nuts, walnuts are second only to peanuts in protein. Black walnuts are especially rich in protein, Vitamin A and E and in iron, phosphorous and magnesium.

WATERCRESS (Naturtium officinale)

Watercress contains more sulphur than any other vegetable except horseradish. In addition to containing certain sulphur bearing amino acids which are necessary for hair growth, it contains valuable amounts of beta carotene, folic acid, biotin, nicotinic acid, pantothenic acid, B1 and lot of C. It is one of the best sources of iodine outside of sea vegetables such as kelp.

Its juice should be mixed with carrot or other juices as it is much too strong to take alone.

WATERMELON (Citrullus vulgaris)

The watermelon rind, the green and white layers between the outside skin and the red centre, is said to contain the richest proteins, vitamins, enzymes and minerals. The green layer immediately beneath the skin contains chlorophyll which makes it easily digestible, even to those who might otherwise have difficulty with melons. The watermelon is especially good in flushing out the whole urinary tract, the bladder and the kidneys and helps dissolve hard deposits which may have come from an inadequate diet. It also helps keep the body on the alkaline side.

BOOK REVIEWS

What has amazed me throughout my quest with cancer, is the hunger and passion I have had to acquire more knowledge about this degenerative disease. In all of my years, I have never been one to sit and read a book, let alone be engrossed in it.

I must say I was fortunate to have been led by some brilliant people which helped me achieve my goals in life. I kept myself educated and 'up to date' with our changing world, by doing business with many successful and educated people. Unlike so many people who do not want to hear the 'C' word let alone talk about it, I was even more determined to learn as much as possible about it. The way our body works, how the cancer cells form, all the different types of cancer and so forth and most especially the cures for cancer.

From reading my first book about cancer which was "A Cancer Therapy" by Dr Max Gerson, I have branched out to other books which in turn have kept leading me to many other informative books, from psychological, spiritual, nutritional to relaxation.

I would like to outline in brief several books which I have found to be most informative and helpful. Most of the books I have been able to purchase from Cope Book Shop at 116 Hutt Street,

Adelaide, South Australia. Tel: 08 8223 3433. Check with a bookstore in your area for availability of books. They should be able to order them in for you if they are not in stock. Or you can contact the internet bookstore, Amazon.com.

Beyond any first and second opinions that may be offered, there are other options that you may wish to consider. The following books will offer you the opportunity to learn about these options so that you can make a truly informed decision.

I would like to start off my book reviews with none other than my life saving book:

A Cancer Therapy, Results of Fifty Cases
5th Edition © 1990 by the Gerson Institute
(Ed. Gar Hildenbrand). ISBN 0-88268-105-2

Dr Max Gerson, MD, was born in Wongrowitz Germany in 1881. It was upon suffering severe migraines, that led him to the now famous 'Gerson Therapy'. From helping patients with his new 'migraine diet' he soon realised it was curing patients with tuberculosis and then cancer. In his book you will find the complete guide to the therapy and results of fifty cured cases, together with photos of X-rays.

When reading this book and many of those listed, I would recommend the purchase of a medical dictionary to assist in deciphering the medical terms. I found this book inspirational and felt the spirit of Max Gerson alive within these pages.

"I could not believe that reading one book could save my life!"

Dr Lorraine Day's Video

In Dr Day's video you will be :

- Guided to a variety of effective therapies documented in the medical literature but rarely revealed to the public.
- Why people get cancer.
- How to get well without vomiting and losing your hair.
- Cancer is Big Business.
- Who controls the cancer business and why effective and safe cancer therapies available 50 years ago have been suppressed.
- How you can control whether you get sick or stay well and how to avoid buying cancer at the store.

It was upon viewing her video that I learnt more about other alternative therapies and different literature to read. To order any of her videos or books, see the order form at the back of the book.

I would like to expand my summary on her by giving you a little insight on her life as reprinted from "The Gerson Healing Newsletter", Vol.10, Number 1, Jan-Feb 1995.

Dr Lorraine Day has impressive credentials. She is an internationally acclaimed orthopedic trauma surgeon and author. She was for 15 years on the faculty of the University of California, San Francisco, School of Medicine as Associate Professor and Vice Chairman of the Department of Orthopedics. She was also Chief of Orthopedic Surgery at San Francisco General Hospital and is recognised world-wide as an AIDS expert. She has been invited to lecture extensively throughout the U.S. and the world; appeared on numerous radio and television shows, including 60 Minutes, Nightline, CNN Crossfire, Oprah Winfrey and Larry King Live.

Dr Lorraine Day has the courage to defy orthodox medicine by getting up before the entire audience of the Cancer Control Society and testifying, as follows:

"I am Dr Lorraine Day. Some of you know me from my book I wrote AIDS–What the Government Isn't Telling You. Several years ago, I actually spoke here about AIDS. I have been coming to the Cancer Control Society meetings regularly for three years and I have learned more about medicine and how to take care of yourself than I learned in 20 years as an orthodox trauma surgeon. I knew nothing about nutrition as a medical doctor. In the four years of medical school, you don't have one single hour of information on nutrition. I have talked about that and admitted that I, in the past, have told patients that their nutrition has really nothing to do with their health. I was ignorant, I was stupid as many orthodox medical doctors are. Fortunately, I found out what was really going on in the health field by coming to the Cancer Control Society, and I started speaking out about it, studying it and actually had a radio show called "Truth Serum" where I was interviewing many alternative doctors. In the middle of that, I found out that I had breast cancer. I had infiltrating ductal carcinoma and it was spreading through my breast.

I went to my first doctor to have the lump taken out. At that time I did not know it was cancer. He refused to take care of me unless I had pre-operative chemotherapy. Even though I told him that I was a physician, and that I would sign any papers releasing him from any legal liability — but that I didn't want chemotherapy. I just wanted the lump taken out and diagnosed. He said No. His reputation was at stake. So, I walked out of his office realising that the law considers it acceptable for a physician to abandon a patient if the patient refuses the doctor's prescription. So I went to a former resident colleague, who is a breast cancer surgeon. He took the lump out but he couldn't get all the cancer. He said, 'You don't have your breast removed, you must have radiation therapy.' Once again, I declined. Then he said, 'You must have chemotherapy or some other kind of treatment to destroy these cancer cells.' I told him 'No, I brought you a whole stack of books, if you really want to learn about cancer, read these books. I won't have any of the orthodox treatments — just take the lump out.' He said that he could not get all the cancer. I said, 'Fine. Everybody gets cancer all the time. My body can take care of that!'

I immediately went home and called up Marilyn Barnes, whom you just heard earlier. (Marilyn Barnes had just previously testified to her total recovery, now over 14 years, from stage 4 melanoma as well as carcinoma in situ-cervical cancer on the Gerson Therapy.) Marilyn came to my house and set me up. She taught a woman I hired how to do the Gerson Therapy. The Gerson Therapy was going to be the basis of my treatment. I started the juices, the enemas, the whole business. In fact, I looked at cancer as a great adventure. Unfortunately, I didn't have the time to take all the different alternatives, but I tried as many as I could. But the Gerson Diet is the basis of all my treatment.

"I am fine. I am healthy. I don't have any evidence of cancer".

Dr Lorraine Day has recently released another video describing the exact plan she used to get well.

To order: See order form in back of book.

Third Opinion
Author: John M. Fink
Publisher: Avery Publishing Group. ISBN 0-89529-503-2

This is an international directory to alternative therapy centres for the treatment and prevention of cancer and other degenerative diseases. It is a comprehensive guide to the many alternative treatment centres located throughout the world. Everything from addresses, phone numbers, names, prices, to philosophical approaches and methods of treatment is provided in a clear, easy to use format. Also included are educational centres, information services and support groups throughout the world. To further help you, the author has included a glossary of terms, a regional breakdown of centres, and a list of informative readings.

The author, John M. Fink, had been an actor for fourteen years when he lost his daughter to cancer. Since then, he has been deeply interested in alternative and adjunctive care. He has been active as a board member of the International Association of Cancer Victors and Friends, both nationally and in the Santa Barbara Chapter. He has also been on the Advisory Board of the National Health Federation, and has served as a member of the Advisory Panel for the Congressional Office of Technology Assessment's study, Unorthodox Cancer

Treatments: Information, Evaluation, and Policy. He resides in Southern California with his wife and two children.

Options (The Alternative Cancer Therapy Book)
Author: Richard Walters
Publisher: Avery Publishing Group Inc. ISBN 0-89529-510-5

This is a most informative and well explained book on alternative therapies. It contains the names, addresses and phone numbers of clinics thoughout the world. It particularly specifies which therapy is appropriate for a specific cancer. This eliminates the time spent on pursuing a therapy which may not assist your particular cancer.

Cancer and Vitamin C
Author: Ewan Cameron and Linus Pauling
© 1979, 1993 Linus Pauling Institute of Science & Medicine
Publisher: Camino Books Inc. ISBN 0-940159-21-X

Linus Pauling, PhD, is a research professor and founder of the Linus Pauling Institute of Science and Medicine. He won the Nobel Prize for chemistry in 1954 and for Peace in 1963.

Ewan Cameron, MB, ChB, FRCS, (Edinburgh and Glasgow) was Director at the Linus Pauling Institute of Science and Medicine. I found this book to be very informative and exciting. I could not believe that a simple vitamin such as Vitamin C which is readily available, can in the correct dosage, help cure cancer.

The book provides helpful details on dosage and methods of administration. It also covers various modes of treatment:

surgery, radiation, chemotherapy, hormones, immunotherapy and a number of unorthodox ones. *"Very informative!"*

Two books which expose the disturbing facts about our drinking water are: "The Water You Drink" and "Fluoride, The Ageing Factor"

The Water You Drink

Author: John Archer, © 1996
Publisher: Pure Water Press. ISBN 0-646-26524-5

This is the most helpful and informative book yet written about Australian drinking water. John Archer is an author, researcher and consumer advocate with a passionate interest in water issues. It covers topics from local and imported waters to water purification in the home and office. It contains a list of suppliers of domestic water treatment and equipment as a service to readers. It also outlines the following topics:

- Lead in first flush tap water
- Chlorine-resistant viruses and parasites
- Aluminium and Alzheimer's disease
- Bladder cancer and chlorination by-products
- Blue green algal toxins and illness
- Herbicide, metabolites and genetic damage
- Tap water, infertility and sexual dysfunction

"A must read book for all Australians concerned about their children's drinking water."

Fluoride, The Ageing Factor

Author: Dr John Yiamouyiannis, BS, PhD, © 1993

Publisher: Health Action Press. ISBN 0-913571-03-2.

This publication delves into the subject of fluoridation in water.

Dr John Yiamouyiannis received his BS in Biochemistry from the University of Chicago and his PhD in Biochemistry from the University of Rhode Island. After completing post doctoral research at Western Reserve University Medical School, he became a biochemist editor at Chemical Abstracts Service, the world's largest chemical information centre where he first became aware of the health-damaging effects of fluoride.

Dr Yiamouyiannis is a world-leading authority on the biological effects of fluoride. Even the American Dental Association cautions its fluoridation speakers, "Running up against Yiamouyiannis is not recommended." He has appeared on national television shows for ABC, CNN, and CNBC. He has spoken before audiences throughout the United States, as well as in Canada, Great Britain, Australia, Japan and Brazil

Responsible for stopping fluoridation in the US and abroad, he notes,"With truth as an ally, it's a lot easier to win. The truth is, fluoridation is chronically poisoning millions".

Nutrition Almanac

Author: Lavon J. Dunne, ©

Publisher: McGraw-Hill Publishing Co. ISBN 0-07-034912-6

The Nutrition Almanac contains:

- An important new study of drinking water.
- Information regarding the sources and dosage levels of vitamins and mineral supplements.
- The latest information about herbs and herbal preparations.
- An easy-to-read food composition chart, providing a nutrition analysis of over 600 foods.
- A complete cooking guide for healthier eating, with recipes.

"I found it to be an excellent reference guide".

Organic Gardening
Author: Peter Bennett. ISBN 1-86436-043-7

Organic gardening is the skill of growing both ornamental and food plants using only natural fertilisers and pest control methods. Every day more Australians are becoming concerned about the long term effects of chemical fertilisers and pesticides, not only upon people, but upon all living things, in the food chains of the world. Peter Bennett has been successfully gardening using traditional methods for over 40 years with outstanding results and Organic Gardening, has become an accepted major work on the subject. This fully revised edition includes over 70 new colour photographs.

The book is an extremely useful and practical guide to all aspects of growing and cultivating plants using natural methods. The text is clear and instructive and is well supported with line drawings and photographs.

Peter Bennett is a journalist, broadcaster, specialist lecturer and professional consultant in alternative horticulture and agricultural ecology. Peter has been a guest lecturer at Macquarie, Sydney, Latrobe and Hobart Universities and has become well known in both Australia and New Zealand.

Today, Peter and his wife Sandra conduct a professional consultancy service, Adult Education courses at the Organic Garden and Farm Service and Supply Centre in Adelaide.

Root Canal Cover-Up

Author: George E. Meinig, DDS, FACD, © 1994
Publisher: Bion Publishing. ISBN 0-945196-19-9

Dr George E. Meinig was one of a very few, who first treated root canal infections and was one of the founding members who started the American Association of Endodontists (root canal therapists). He has had a life time experience in the field and worked in many places and written for many papers, from Managing the Twentieth Century Fox Studio dental clinic to 17 years of writing in the Ojai Valley News. Along his working life he came to learn about the 25 year root canal research of Dr Weston Price and the serious effects which can result.

In his book he goes through the work of Dr Weston Price in which he uncovers the infections of organ, glands and tissues caused by bacteria trapped inside the structure of teeth. These infected organs or tissues can in turn, damage the heart, kidneys, joints, eyes, brain and endanger pregnant women. After 47 years of being an experienced dentist and root canal therapist, Dr George E. Meinig was indeed amazed and interested to see the connection between the infected tooth and disease.

"It is time for dentists and patients to realise the decay of teeth is not just a local disturbance but is actually a systemic disease involving the whole body."

Two books which recount a personal battle and victory over cancer are "Cancer Winner" and "A Time to Heal". I found "A Cancer Winner" truly inspirational and whenever feeling a little low, I would immediately turn to those pages and feel invigorated.

A Cancer Winner

Author: Jaquie Davison, © 1977
Publisher: Midwest Press
PO Box 159, Pierce City MO 65723 USA

Within these pages you will travel along the road of battle to 'Victory' with Jaquie. She is truly a woman to be admired for her strength and courage.

Jaquie was diagnosed with malignant melanoma in August 1974 and her cancer grew persistently until August 1975. She was only 38-years-old and had eight children and a devoted husband. Within the year of diagnosis, she tried several recommended health cures after she had refused the standard chemotherapy and radiation, but none seemed to help. She accepted her fate and prepared for her death, even sewing her own burial dress. It was while she was deteriorating and waiting for death, that her husband gave her Dr Max Gerson's book "A Cancer Therapy".

She started living her new life and has now been in remission for over 20 years from Stage 4 melanoma.

Both Anna and myself highly recommend this book for enlightenment and courage.

A Time to Heal
Author: Beata Bishop, © 1985
Publisher: Severn House Publishers Ltd in Great Britain.
ISBN 0-450-50085-3

Beata Bishop is a writer and psychotherapist. She has worked as a journalist and spent 11 years writing radio scripts for the BBC. It was around November 1979 when undergoing a routine check up, that she was diagnosed with melanoma on her leg. After a year and part of her leg mutilated by surgery, she was again diagnosed with secondary cancer around June 1981. She was given six months to live and she was also suffering at this time with incipient osteo-arthritis, diabetes, migraines, and chronic dental abscesses. After orthodox medicine had very little to offer her, she turned to alternative medicine and the Gerson Therapy.

For 18 months she travelled from the edge of death to a more abundant life. Not only did she overcome her cancer but all her other ailments as well. Doctors and friends assured her that regeneration of her mutilated leg was impossible and she believed them — only she happened to be walking on that impossibility everyday, as a large part of that same mutilated leg had grown back. You will travel with her through her journey from life-threatening disease to health.

Another book that will show you that where there is love and belief, there is survival and inner peace.

The Cure For All Cancers
Author: Hulda Regehr Clark, PhD, ND
Publisher: New Century Press.

New research findings show there is a single cause for all cancers. This book provides exact instructions for their cure and also includes over 100 case histories of persons cured.

"A truly amazing book".

The Human Body
Author: Gillian Bunce
Publisher: © Struik Publishers Pty Ltd. ISBN 1-85368-355-8

The reason I chose this book is because it gives a simple informative introduction to the human body.

"This type of book will help you 'to read your body'.

The following books helped me to strengthen my most vital asset — MY MIND.

Life Without Stress

Author: Ainslie Meares

Publisher: Viking O'Neil Penguin Books Australia.

ISBN 0 -670-90359-0

Ainslie Meares was a man of great eminence. Foundation Fellow of the Royal Australian and New Zealand College of Psychiatrists and past President of the International Society for Clinical and Experimental Hypnosis, he was an international authority on hypnosis. He worked for thirty years as a psychiatrist and used meditation extensively in the treatment of psycho neurotic and psychosomatic illnesses. In 1976, in the *Medical Journal of Australia*, he first reported on the regression of cancer following intensive meditation. This step away from orthodox medicine's cancer regime of chemotherapy, radiotherapy and surgery brought him into direct conflict with the medical profession. However, in 1981 *The Lancet* published his findings on regression of cancer in the absence of any orthodox treatment and eventually his meditative techniques were accepted by the medical profession with the exception of oncologists.

Dr Meares was the author of thirty books on both technical and popular aspects of psychiatry, including the best-seller "Relief Without Drugs" and its update "The Wealth Within". His books have been translated into seven languages. Dr Meares died in September 1986.

Relief Without Drugs

Author: Ainslie Meares

Publisher: Angus & Robertson. ISBN 0207-18898X

Dr Meares describes in detail the simple techniques he advocates to relieve pain and strain, both mental and physical. He gives the case histories of patients who have overcome their disabilities and found themselves able to face life with renewed strength and hope.

The Wealth Within

Author: Ainslie Meares

Publisher: Hill of Content. ISBN 0-85572-086-7

This is a self-help book which takes the reader through a step-by-step course of global relaxation so that a state of Mental Ataraxis, or freedom from disturbance, is achieved.

The method described veers away from other forms of meditational relaxation in that it is global — not progressive — and requires a posture of discomfort rather than comfort in order to allow the relaxation to come from the mind, not the body. Restoration occurs at the deepest centre of being. In achieving the state of Mental Ataraxis, there is the attainment of an inner stillness — a moment of complete freedom from disturbance — whereby the natural restorative activities of mind and body, including the natural immune system of the body, are regenerated.

The book includes a section which explains how the regular practice of Mental Ataraxis will improve the quality of life. With the shedding of tension and anxiety there is immediate improvement in the quality of life experienced at work, at leisure, in the home and in inter-personal relationships including sexual relationships.

Peace of Mind

Author: Dr Ian Gawler

Publisher: Hill of Content. ISBN 0-85572-167-7

Meditation's ultimate goal is to generate peace of mind. In the process it produces many other tangible benefits. Meditation can transform your life. This best selling classic clearly and completely sets out the many benefits and techniques of meditation. This information is presented in a style that combines the clear logic of the western intellect with the intuitive insight of the eastern mystic.

This is an outstanding book by an author who is an authority on meditation and mind power. Scientific evidence is confirming the paramount importance of the mind in the cause and treatment of illness.

You Can Conquer Cancer

Author: Ian Gawler

Publisher: Hill of Content. ISBN 0-88572-141-3

The best selling self-help classic on the prevention and management of cancer.

Instant Calm

Author: Paul Wilson

Publisher: Penguin Books. ISBN 0-14-024494-8

Here clearly described, are over a hundred of the most powerful calming techniques known, from the wisdom of ancient civilisations to the discoveries of modern research.

When I first started my 'Cancer Crusade', I had two very disturbing questions that needed to be answered.

1. *"Why on earth would our medical establishment try to suppress a cure for cancer?"*
2. *"Don't you think if there were a cure for cancer, our medical establishment would have told us?"*

The following reviews answer these two questions.

The Cancer Industry

The Classic Expose On The Cancer Establishment

Author: Ralph W. Moss, PhD

Publisher: Equinox Press, New York. ISBN 1-881025-09-8

"Everyone should know that the 'War on Cancer' is largely a fraud". — Linus Pauling PhD, and two times nobel prize winner.

When President Nixon declared 'war on cancer' in 1971, leading scientists promised Congress a cure in time for the Bicentennial. That didn't happen, and almost everyone agrees that overall, the results of the war on cancer have been meagre. Something is terribly wrong and this book attempts to tell why.

Racketeering in Medicine – The Suppression of Alternatives
Author: Dr James P. Carter
Publisher: Hampton Roads Publishing Company Inc.
ISBN 1-878901-32-X

Can we assume that our health is always the prime concern of organized medicine? Or are we being deprived of effective, economical treatments because those treatments are not highly profitable for surgeons and pharmaceutical companies?

Dr Carter does not speak in generalities or put forth vague accusations. He presents names, events and facts of interest to all concerned, and leads the reader to the inescapable realisation that we must become more aware of health care practices and speak up for our right to the best available medical treatment.

The Chemotherapy Survival Guide
Author: Judith McKay, RN and Nancee Hirano, RN, MSN
Publisher: New Harbinger Publications, Inc.
ISBN 1-879237-57-1

If you are facing chemotherapy, this book can be both a reference and a comforting voice. It has real answers to many of the important questions you have. It's a self-help book that emphasises what you can do to cope. From blood tests and intravenous medication to dealing with hair loss, nausea, stress, etc., this book is written clearly, candidly, and supportively. It contains many hints and practical suggestions that nurses give their patients, and that you can use to feel more empowered during this time.

"You may forget to ask your specialist certain questions, or feel embarrassed. This book gives answers to many of the most commonly asked questions".

The Australian Drug Guide

Author: Dr Jonathan Upfal © 1995
Printer: Griffin Paperbacks, Adelaide SA. ISBN 186-381-184-2

"The Australian Drug Guide" is the first ever complete reference to drugs that has been written in plain English. Every drug profile includes:

- Chemical name (and how to pronounce it), drug class to which it belongs and all brand names.
- Whether a prescription is required and if the drug is subsidised by the Governments.
- What is it for? How does it work? When you shouldn't take it and special preventions.
- Dosages and strengths, how to take the drug, major and minor side effects.
- Possible long-term side effects and complications.

Hydrogen Peroxide, Medical Miracle

Author: Dr William Campbell Douglass,
Publisher: Second Opinion Publishing. ISBN 1-885236-07-7

Dr William Campbell Douglass is a fourth generation physician. He is a graduate of the University of Rochester, New York; the University of Miami School of Medicine; and the United States Naval School of Aviation and Space Medicine. Dr Douglass travels the world giving lectures, doing radio and TV talk shows and gathering information that is not covered by our press.

Hydrogen Peroxide (H_2O_2) is involved in all of life's vital processes. It is truly the wonder molecule. The cells in the body that fight infection, called granulocytes, produce H_2O_2 as a first line of defense against every type of invading organism — parasites, viruses, bacteria and yeast. The presence of this amazing substance is required for the metabolism of protein, carbohydrates, fats, vitamins, and minerals. It must be present for the immune system to function properly.

The Essiac Report
Author: Richard Thomas
Publisher: The Alternative Treatment Information Network.
1244 Ozeta Terrace, Los Angeles CA 90069 USA
Tel: 1-310-278-6611

This is the true story of a Canadian herbal cancer remedy and of the thousands of lives it continues to save.

Get a Life – The detoxification cure made easy
Author: Kathryn Alexander
Publisher: National Direct Publishing. ISBN 0-646-31829-2
Web: http:/www.getalife.on.net

This is one of the most recent books I have read and found it to be in line with the Gerson methodology. It is very easy to follow and provides an extremely effective detoxification programme.

It offers various detoxification plans and allows the reader to choose which is best suited for them.

Kathryn Alexander is a qualified Dietary Therapist, having attained her qualifications in London. I have had the pleasure of personally meeting Kathryn, and have found her to be a true humanitarian.

I highly recommend this book.

Cancer Leukaemia, The Bruess Cancer Cure
Author: Rudolph Breuss with Hilde Hemmes
Published under License in Australia and New Zealand by:
Australian School of Herbal Medicine © 1997.
ISBN 0-646-34773-X

This book is very easy to read with many testimonials and the actual therapy listed in detail.

CERTIFIED ORGANIC PRODUCE LOCALITY GUIDE

The following information has been reprinted with the kind permission of ORGAA (Organic Retailers & Growers Association of Australia Inc.), PO Box 12852, A'Beckett Street, Melbourne VIC 3000.

In recent years there has been increasing concern over how our food has been produced, how it has been modified during processing and what effect additives and accidental contaminants, such as pesticides may have on our health. Organic food with its stringent production guidelines, has therefore, become increasingly in demand.

Organically grown food is a precise term in that it specifically relates to food that has been grown on a certain kind of farm, using special methods of production. Organic food therefore, presents consumers with a perceived set of attributes that align themselves with environmentally acceptable production techniques which minimise the risk of contamination from pesticides, and also delivers food which is wholesome and nutritious.

Consumers should only buy produce which is clearly identified by a certification logo. These are:

1. BIODYNAMIC AGRICULTURAL ASSOCIATION OF AUSTRALIA

2. BIOLOGICAL FARMERS CO-OPERATIVE LTD

3. NATIONAL ASSOCIATION FOR SUSTAINABLE AGRICULTURE

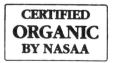

4. ORGANIC HERB GROWERS ASSOCIATION

5. ORGANIC VIGNERONS ASSOCIATION OF AUSTRALIA INC.

Certified Retailers of Australia

Please note that other organic food outlets exist throughout Australia, simply look for them in your telephone book, under 'Organic'.

ALTONA NORTH ORGANICS
Altona North, Victoria
Ph: (03) 9391 3282

BENDIGO HEALTH FOODS
Bendigo, Victoria
Ph: (03) 5441 3542

ORGANIC GREENS AND GRAINS
Prahran, Victoria
Ph: (03) 9510 4256

DON'T PANIC ITS ORGANIC
Mt. Eliza, Victoria
Ph: (03) 9775 2024

DYNAMIC VEGIES ORGANIC FOOD SUPPLY
Eltham, Victoria
Ph: (03) 9439 3462

EASTFIELD NATURAL FOODS
Croydon, Victoria
Ph: (03) 9723 0257

ELWOOD ORGANIC FRUIT
Elwood, Victoria
Ph: (03) 9531 6305

FRUIT PEDALLERS
Northcote, Victoria
Ph: (03) 9489 5824

GARDEN ORGANICS
Stall 85-86 T Shed
Queen Victoria Market, Victoria

GO ORGANIC
Fitzroy
Ph./Fax: (03) 9417 7476

GULLY GREEN GROCER
Ferntree Gully, Victoria
Ph: (03) 9758 8650

JOSEPH'S A1 FRUIT STALL
Shop 12, Fyshwick Market, Fyshwick, ACT

KAGU HEALTH
South Melbourne Market, Victoria
Ph: (03) 9531 1718 Mobile: 0412 311 718

MELBOURNE ORGANICS
South Melbourne, Victoria
Ph: (03) 9690 93390

MELBOURNE ORGANICS
St. Kilda, Victoria
Ph: (03) 9537 0144

MORE HEALTH
Sydney Markets, New South Wales

ORGANIC ACTION
Ph: (02) 9544 6252 or (02) 9746 3105

ORGANIC FOOD BOUTIQUE

43 South Crescent, North Gosford NSW 2250

Ph: 043 257 179

ORGANIC GROCERY

Richmond, Victoria

Ph: (03) 9429 9219

ORGANICALLY GROWN

Malvern, Victoria

Ph: (03) 9500 9796

ORGANICS AT THE MARKET

Melbourne, Victoria

Ph: (03) 9585 7068 Mob: 015 326 694 Fax: (03) 9484 9622

ORGANIC WHOLEFOODS

East Brunswick, Victoria

Ph: (03) 9384 0288 Fax: (03) 9384 1322

ORGANIC WHOLEFOODS

Fitzroy, Victoria

Ph: (03) 9419 5347

RED HILL GREEN GROCER

Red Hill, South Victoria

Ph: (03) 5989 2066

SIMPLY ORGANIC

Frankston, Victoria

Ph / Fax: (03) 5971 4063

THE ENCHANTED BROCCOLI FOREST
Norwood, South Australia
Ph: (08) 8431 0038

WILSON'S ORGANICS
57A Gouger Street, Adelaide, South Australia 5000
Ph: (08) 8231 5014 Fax: (08) 8231 4263

ORGANICALLY GROWN
55B St Bernards Road, Magill, South Australia 5072
Ph: (08) 8364 1699

THE FRIENDLY FOOD CO-OP
Ballarat, Victoria
Ph: (03) 5333 3720

THE GREEN GROCER
North Fitzroy, Victoria

THE GREEN LIME
Hartwell, Victoria
Ph: (03) 9889 2299 Fax: (03) 9889 1399

THE ORGANIC MARKET
Sterling, South Australia
Ph: (08) 8339 4835

THE ORGANIC UNION
Surrey Hills, Victoria
Ph: (03) 9890 1292

THE WADE FAMILY DIST.
Cheltenham, Victoria
Ph: (03) 9583 8754 Fax: (03) 9583 4987

VIC. MARKET ORGANICS
Victoria Markets, Victoria
Ph: (03) 9387 8078

WHOLEFOODS CO-OP
Geelong, Victoria
Ph: (03) 5221 5421 Fax: (03) 5229 8361

ALFALFA HOUSE
Enmore, NSW
Ph: (02) 9519 3374

ANNABEL'S NATURAL FOOD STORE
Crows Nest, NSW
Ph: (02) 9906 6377 Fax: (02) 9906 6378

AVALONS ORGANICS
Avalon, NSW
Ph: (02) 9918 3387 Fax: (02) 9974 5656

BEEHIVE CO.
Lara, Victoria
Ph: (03) 5282 1386

BELMORE MEATS
Balwyn, East Victoria
Ph: (03) 9857 9379

COLES SUPERMARKETS AUSTRALIA
Glen Iris, Victoria
Ph: (03) 9829 5111

COMMONSENSE ORGANICS
Wellington, New Zealand
Ph: (04) 384 3314 Fax: (04) 385 3383

EARTH FOOD STORE
Bondi Beach, NSW
Ph: (02) 9365 5098

GREEN HARVEST
Maleny, QLD
Ph: (075) 4944 676

A HANDFUL OF SENSE
Surry Hills, NSW
Ph: (02) 9319 7306

HURSTBRIDGE ORGANIC FRUIT SHOP
Hurstbridge, Victoria
Ph: (03) 9718 2327

HURSTBRIDGE WHOLEFOOD DELIGHTS
Hurstbridge, Victoria
Ph: (03) 9718 2873

INNER GLOW HEALTH PRODUCTS
PO Box 162, Tewantin, Queensland 4565
Ph: (07) 5449 0600 Fax: (07) 5449 0900

JASPER COFFEE

Collingwood, Victoria

Ph: (03) 9416 1960

KANDI'S BALWYN HEIGHTS FRUIT SUPPLY

North Balwyn, Victoria

Ph: (03) 9857 9333

LAVENDULA ORGANIC PRODUCTS

New Lambton, NSW

Ph / Fax: (04) 952 1951

MANNA WHOLEFOODS

Freemantle, WA

Ph: (09) 335 7995

MT. LAWLEY WHOLEFOODS

Mt. Lawley, Perth WA

Ph: (09) 227 9072

NATURALLY AWARE

Surrey Hills, Victoria

Ph: (03) 9898 3591

ONE EARTH FOODS

Elanora Heights, NSW

Ph: (02) 9970 6113

ORGANIC FRUIT SHOP

Toowoomba, QLD

Ph: (076) 39 1811 Fax: (076) 39 1671

RYE HEALTH STORE

Rye, Victoria

Ph: (03) 5985 4887

SUMMERHILL ORGANIC FRUIT MARKET

Summer Hill, NSW

Ph: (02) 9799 3258

TOTALLY ORGANIC

Nagambie, Victoria

Ph/Fax: (03) 5794 1687

PURELY ORGANICS

Blackburn, Victoria

Ph: (03) 9877 5477

SANTOS TRADING

Byron Bay, NSW

Ph/Fax: (066) 855 685

WOODEND FRUIT MARKET

Woodend, Victoria

Ph: (03) 5427 2223

YAKAPARI ORGANIC FOODS

Yakapari, QLD

Ph: (079) 54 0820 Fax: (079) 54 0708

Check the yellow pages for other organic retailers.

MEDICATION TABLES

As shown in previous chapters, supplemental medication played an important role in the Gerson Therapy together with nutrition and detoxification. Listed below are the names and description of some of the supplements we took:

Acidol Pepsin in capsule form, these are a source of supplemental hydrochloric acid which are taken before meals. Hydrochloric acid is produced within the stomach to aid the digestive process.

Thyroid in tablet form is given to help correct an imbalanced metabolism. (Each tablet was 65mg).

Niacin in tablet form is necessary for the body's energy metabolism and for the synthesis of fatty acids.

B12 Injections (cynocobalamin) given to replenish the liver's store of this particular vitamin which is essential in the synthesis of DNA.

Lugol's solution is used to restore the loss of iodine.

Potassium compound salts are used to restore the imbalance between sodium and potassium levels within the cells. It is made up of potassium gluconate, potassium acetate and mono-potassium phosphate in equal amounts. (33.34gm) of each potassium salt mixed to one litre of water.

Liver Capsules are used to replace liver juice.

Pancreatin in tablet form is taken to aid digestion.

Wobe Mugos and *CoQ10* were two complimentary supplements I took whilst at the Gerson Clinic.

Wobe Mugos is a very powerful digestive enzyme used to compliment the overall therapy. Each tablet contains Papain 100mg, Trypsin 40mg and Chymotrypsin 40mg. These are not readily available in Australia so it would be necessary to consult with a health practitioner.

CoQ10 has a direct affect on the cells energy level production and is readily available from your local health store.

Triad consists of 50mg niacin, 500mg ascorbic acid (vitamin C) and a 300mg aspirin.

Germanium is a potent immune enhancing mineral. Organic Germanium is a prevalent trace mineral element that acts as a semi-conductor, entering into our bio-chemical equations by balancing the oxygen content of the cells — an 'oxygen carrier'. It's proper name is Bis-betacarboxyethyl germanium sesquioxide, and as a mineral, it helps conduct the body bioelectricity. It is a clear to white crystalline, odourless powder.

The key activity of germanium appears to be the added oxygenation made available by the special sesquioxide chemistry, wherein three oxygen molecules are readily available for the oxidation mechanisms. Dr Kazuhiko Asai, a Japanese chemist, perfected a process of producing crystalline germanium, after finding the highest concentrations of it in medicinal plants. He says he cured his own advanced arthritis with it, by taking 250 to 1,500mg/day orally. He also states that, when the blood is too acidic, germanium is not effective. It is produced by: MONARCH LABORATORIES, Ogden Utah, 84401 USA.

PREDICTIONS

"The energy required to have the will to survive is in proportion to the energy required to search for that will."

The following predictions are based on my own personal observations and experience. I envisage these changes occurring within the next five years.

1. Every home in Australia will have a reservoir of water on their premises, as a rainwater tank, a bore, or an in-house water distillation system. This won't arise because of lack of water, but because of its degenerative quality. Fluoride and chlorine will no longer be added to our water supplies. These toxic substances will not be tolerated by the public. They will be replaced with non-toxic methods of purification. eg. Ozone and Hydrogen Peroxide as currently used in some US states.

2. All dentists will no longer use mercury amalgams, nor will root canal procedures continue to be used. Once the public become aware of just how devastating these procedures are, they will soon disappear from dental clinics.

3. Butchers and greengrocers will sell only certified organic / free range produce.

4. In addition to current orthodox cancer therapies, the medical profession will be required to send their patients to counselling and nutrition courses.

5. Pharmacies will carry health products such as vitamins and herbs which will require prescriptions.

6. Most fast food outlets will be replaced by health cafes and juice bars, with an emphasis on nutritious, well balanced, living foods. This will occur because of the growing awareness within the community of the health benefits of wholesome living food.

7. Due to the diminishing nutritional content in conventional fruits and vegetables, people will start growing their own produce. Back yards will be transformed into colourful vegetable gardens, artistically created, so as to maintain practicality and beauty.

8. Many more professionals within the orthodox medical industry, will incorporate alternative medicine within their practices. This will happen for a number of reasons. Some of these are already apparent today.

   a) Doctors, together with other health professionals, will need to expand their knowledge of Alternative Therapies to survive financially.

   b) The growing awareness within the community of the positive effects of alternative medicine.

c) Alternative medicine is now becoming more widely accepted by the community. This is due in part, to our multi-cultural society, ie. Chinese and Indian medicine.

d) Many are becoming frustrated with orthodox medicine because it simply masks the real problem and doesn't address the cause.

9. The role of veterinary surgeons will change, whereby they will assist in determining specific diets, not only for animals but also for humans. They will also help to diagnose the causes of specific diseases so as to prescribe their treatment.

TO OUR GENETIC IMMORTALITY

To our wondrous children who have brought into our lives love, laughter, tears, joy, wisdom, and a warm fuzzy feeling.

I would like to pass onto you the knowledge we have attained which only comes with the experience of having made many mistakes.

- May your Angel help you to enhance and preserve your sense of LOGIC, your OBSERVATION skills and your COMMON SENSE. These are Survival Skills.

- Be as COURAGEOUS as the Men and Women who unselfishly and unconditionally gave their lives to protect the land in which we now live.

- Travel the world so you may appreciate what you currently take for granted.

- Don't be misguided into believing all you see or hear.

- ASK QUESTIONS. It's the only way you will get answers. And once you get the answer, ask yourself the same question.

- Meditate, pray or just relax on a daily basis.

- Before trusting your judgement, take 10 minutes to think about it. This will add to your wisdom.

- Be free with this life, don't get too attached to materialistic objects. You can't take them with you.

- Be self sufficient, grow your own organic fruits and vegetables.

- Learn to play a musical instrument. This is the universal language.

- Learn to play a sport. This will help you to develop your physical and mental strengths.

- Learn to speak another language.

- Be creative, be different. You're not sheep.

- Keep your leadership qualities with you always. This will help create credibility.

- Be courteous and helpful, especially to children and the elderly. They have the wisdom.

- Work, exercise and rest on a daily basis.

- AVOID drugs of any type, including tobacco smoking and alcohol. These are soul destructive.

- Get high on conversation, laughter, music, sport, and adventure.

- Learn to cook, using nature to enhance the flavours. Avoid salt, sugar, and anything artificial.

- By eating the correct foods you will eliminate any Inherited Genetic Burden (IGB) onto yourself and your children.

- Do not look at yourself as a mass, but as a single cell. A cell that will keep you alive if you feed it correctly.

- Do not fear to ask. If you do not ask the fear remains.

- In times of need, ask your angel of hope.

- Reduce time spent on the Relaxation Inhibiting Devices (RID)
  1. *Telephone*
  2. *Television*
  3. *Personal pager*
  4. *Radio*
  5. *Computer*

- Replace panic with Prayer and fear with Faith.

- The best way to learn is from other peoples mistakes.

- If you feel tired then rest.
  If you are thirsty then drink.
  If you feel hungry then eat.
  These are fundamental requirements for 'Body Listening'.

- One deep breath is worth 10 shallow.

- Study the human anatomy so you can fine tune your listening abilities.

- Don't preach. Speak only to those that thirst to know.

- PATIENCE IS THE ESSENCE OF THE SOUL.

- Respect all religions and cultures.

- Visit the cancer ward of a Children's Hospital.

- Be quiet and still. Learn to listen.

- Be versed in medicine and law.

- Love, respect and help one another.

- Every morning upon you wake, SMILE, for goodness sake.

- BELIEVE IN ANGELS

. . . Love Mum and Dad.

SAYINGS OF 'GRANDPA THORNBURG'

I would like to share with you some sayings that were passed onto us whilst in Mexico. Written by 'Grandpa Thornburg':

"A smile adds a great deal to your face value"
"Advice is like castor oil, easy to give but dreadful to take'
"The mind is a bad thing to waste"
"When all think alike, no one thinks very much"
"Treat your friends like family and your family like friends"
"If you refuse to accept anything but the best, you very often get it"
"Horse sense naturally dwells in a stable mind"
"Live for today, plan for tomorrow, and the future will take care of itself"

"Whoever has a heart full of love always has something to give"
"How a little peace of mind can go a long way"
"Let's give thanks that our mirrors can't laugh"
"Horsepower was much safer when only horses had it"

Accompanying the above quotes, was the following letter:

LETTER FROM A WEST VIRGINIAN MOTHER TO HER SON IN VIRGINIA:

Dear Son,

I am writing this slow because I know you can't read fast. We don't live where we did when you left. Your Dad read in the newspaper where most accidents happened within 20 miles of home so we moved. I won't be able to send you the address 'cause the last family that lived here took the numbers with them for their next house so they wouldn't have to change their address.

This place has a washing machine. The first day I put 4 shirts in it, pulled the chain and haven't seen them since. It only rained twice this week. 3 days the first time and 4 days the second time.

The coat you wanted me to send you, Aunt Sarah said it would be a little too heavy to send in the mail with them heavy buttons, so we cut them off and put them in the pockets.

We got a bill from the funeral home, said if we didn't make the last payment on Grandma's funeral bill, up she comes.

About your Father — he has a lovely new job. He has 500 men under him. He is cutting grass at the cemetery.

About your sister — she had a baby this morning. I haven't found out whether it's a boy or girl, so I don't know if you are an aunt or an uncle.

Three of your friends went off the bridge in a pick- up. One was driving — the other two were in the back. The driver got out — he rolled down the window and swam to safety. The other two drowned. They couldn't get the tailgate down.

Your Uncle John fell in the whiskey vat. Some men tried to pull him out, but he fought them off, so he drowned. We cremated him — he burned for 3 days.

Not much more news this time, nothing much happened. Write more often.

Love, Mom

PS. I was going to send you some money, but the envelope was already sealed.

I invite you to share an anecdote or quotation you feel should appear in a future edition. Just send a copy to:

Living Proof
PO Box 377
Magill SOUTH AUSTRALIA 5072
Tel: (08) 8364 4925

EPILOGUE

I would like to end this book by not ending it. What I mean by this is that I would like to invite you, to participate in helping me produce the next book, as a lead on from this. I would like the next book to be based on testimonials.

If you have or had cancer, or know someone, and would like to share with us your story, regarding your experiences with therapies, support groups, nutrition or any other treatments, please write to us regarding you story and send to the address below. Any information will be confidential if requested, and can be submitted without a name if desired. Such information could be an invaluable service to people searching for assistance.

Living Proof
PO Box 377
Magill SOUTH AUSTRALIA 5072

Most of the literature featured here can be ordered from: Inner Glow Products, 77 Pound Road, Warrandyte VIC 3113. Tel: (03) 9844 4471. *See the booking form attached.*

Our Most Popular Books & Videotapes

A Cancer Therapy — Results of Fifty Cases $19.95
Max Gerson, M.D.

The most complete book on the Gerson Therapy. Dr. Gerson explains that the treatment reactivates the body's healing mechanism in chronic degenerative diseases. Extensive explanation of the theory, research and exact practice of the therapy, and presentation of fifty documented case histories. Also included is a modified version of the therapy for use with non-malignant diseases.

Censured for Curing Cancer: The American Experience of Dr. Max Gerson $6.95
S.J. Haught

Newspaper reporter S. J. Haught was assigned to write an article, "The Unveiling of a Quack", about Dr. Gerson. This book is Haught's story of his research, and his own discovery of Gerson's success in healing "incurable" illness. The book has many personal stories, and examines the suppression of information about Gerson's treatment. Also included are case histories, and Dr. Gerson's 1946 testimony before the U.S. Senate, in which he presented healed "incurable" cancer patients.

The Gerson Primer $19.95
Edited by the Gerson Institute

A companion to A Cancer Therapy, this handbook is provided to each patient at Gerson Therapy Centers. The Gerson Primer provides a detailed discussion of procedures at the hospital, and includes notes from lectures by hospital physicians, adjuvant therapies and procedures, necessities for doing the therapy at home, laboratory test interpretation and more. Includes all of the recipes in the Gerson Therapy Recipe book.

Gerson Therapy Recipes. $5.95
Edited by the Gerson Institute

A variety of delicious, healthy recipes — main courses, side dishes, desserts and salads — for Gerson Therapy patients and anyone who wants to heal and prevent disease through diet. A companion to the Food Preparation video.

A Time to Heal (formerly My Triumph Over Cancer). $12.95
Beata Bishop

Told that her spreading melanoma would take her life by 1981, Beata traveled from London to Mexico to begin Gerson Therapy treatment. She writes about her experiences at the hospital with humor and introspection. Beata is an experienced journalist and broadcaster for the BBC, and her book illustrates her newfound sense of well being.

The Gerson Healing Newsletters $65.00
The complete set of 48 back issues of the membership publication of the Gerson Institute. Includes many interesting articles, case histories of recovered patients, and scientific rationales for various aspects of the Gerson therapy.

The Genial Seed $2.00
Giuliano Dego

An epic 37 stanza poem by one of Europe's foremost poets, a former Gerson patient. A touching, beautiful tribute to Dr. Max Gerson on the centennial of his birth.

Related Books

Fats that Heal, Fats that Kill . $22.95
Udo Erasmus

The most complete guide to fats and oils in health and nutrition, this book describes the success of Dr. Johanna Budwig in using unrefined flax oils to help heal cancer, arteriosclerosis and other degenerative diseases. Important information for Gerson patients and all people.

Fluoride: The Aging Factor . . $14.95
John Yiamouyiannis, Ph.D.

Complete, well-documented research on the use of fluoride in drinking water, toothpaste, and dental treatments. Contrary to popular notion, Yiamouyiannis, a former public health official, shows that fluoride does not reduce cavities, and instead, contributes to mottling of teeth, osteoporosis, cancer, arthritis, and other degenerative diseases.

The Root Canal Coverup $19.95
George Meinig, D.D.S., F.A.C.O.

The founder of the Association of Root Canal Specialists reveals his research into the degenerative diseases and health problems caused by root canals.

Pottinger's Cats $7.95
Frances M. Pottinger, Jr., M.D.

The classic research study showing the dramatic degeneration of successive generations of animals fed cooked food instead of raw food.

Doctor Max $24.95
Giuliano Dego

The story of pioneering physician Max Gerson's acclaimed cancer therapy and his heroic struggle to change the way we look at health and healing. 767 pages.

USE THIS ORDER FORM

to order materials from Dr. Lorraine Day
BOOKS, VIDEOS AND AUDIOS

		QTY.	TOTAL
You Can't Improve on God! (video)	$19.95		
"Cancer Doesn't Scare Me Anymore" (video)	$19.95		
AIDS: What the Government Isn't Telling You (book)	$17.95		
Doctors of Deceit (book by Gus Sermos)	$ 9.95		
Everything you want to know about AIDS but haven't been told (2 video set)			
Video #1	$19.95		
Video #2	$19.95		
Set (Vol. 1&2)	$29.95		
Condoms Don't Work (book)	$10.00		
Can Mosquitoes Transmit AIDS (book)	$10.00		
	Subtotal		
	Sales tax 7.75% CA residents only		
	Shipping and Handling charges (on goods only) SEE CHART BELOW		
	TOTAL		

To order by telephone call toll-free **1-800-574-2437**
To order by mail: send check, money order (U.S. funds only) or credit card number to:

ROCKFORD PRESS
P.O. BOX 8
THOUSAND PALMS, CA 92276

FAX: 1-760-343-0765

Card Number _____

Expiration Date _____

Signature _____

Name _____

Street _____

City _____ State _____

Phone _____ Zip _____

Most orders will be received by customer within 7-10 days.
But, please allow 4 to 6 weeks for delivery.

*Shipping costs MUST be included for order processing.

Shipping & Handling Charges within the U.S.

Under $25:	$4.50
$25 - $34.99:	$6.25
$35 - $49.99:	$7.25
$50 - $74.99:	$8.75
$75 - $99.99:	$9.95
$100 - and up:	add 10%

"Let your angel be your guide"

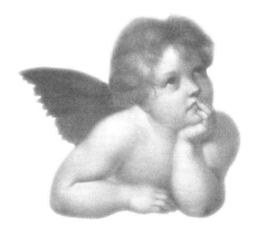